YOGA

TOP 100 YOGA POSES WITH PICTURES

TABLE OF CONTENTS

INTRODUCTION

I want to thank you and congratulate you for downloading the book, "YOGA: Top 100 Poses with Pictures".

For thousands of years, people in India have been practicing yoga to improve the health of the mind, body, and spirit. This ancient practice is known as Hatha Yoga. This is a meditative exercise that makes use of flexible body movements and poses in rechanneling energy for better physical and mental strength, and healing.

Yoga is an optimal form of exercise and can be practiced by any person of any age and race. It is a relaxed yet powerful method of boosting the body's immunity, strength, flexibility, and internal health. It is also an effective way of relieving stress and tension because it relaxes the body and promotes peace of mind.

Yoga is also a cognitive booster. It helps treat anxiety, depression, and other stress-related psychological conditions. And because yoga is a challenging art, it enhances the mind's ability to focus better, think more clearly, and overcome fear.

Aside from being a meditative exercise that promotes health and well-being, yoga is also known to be a therapeutic regimen. Yoga is now popularly practiced as part of alternative therapies for people who are recovering from various physical conditions and those suffering from traumatic psychological disorders.

Thanks again for downloading this book, I hope you enjoy it!

CHAPTER 1

STANDING POSES

Standing poses improves strength. These poses also promote stability and balance, as well as rejuvenate and heal different body parts.

These poses are often used as warm up exercises to prepare the body for a more intense exercise. Any standing pose can be a base for many other poses because it allows easy shifting to more complex poses for meditation and work-out. Furthermore, standing poses improves and establishes work-out posture, so you can proceed without the risk of injuring yourself due to improper body posture.

1. TADASANA OR MOUNTAIN POSE

The Mountain Pose helps improve one's posture, strengthen the inner legs, firm the core, and relieve leg pains.

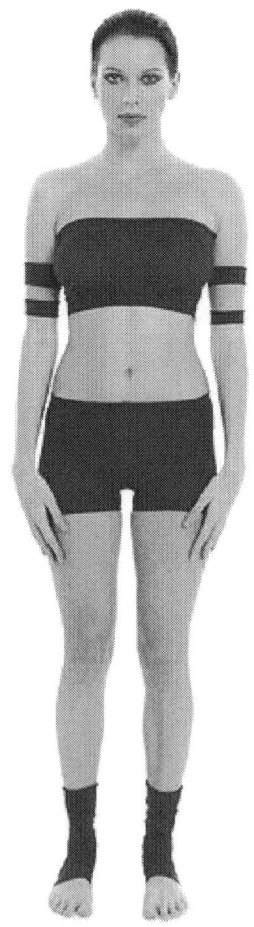

Photo Source: Wikipedia.org

2. VRKSASANA OR TREE POSE

The Tree pose helps improve balance, strengthen leg muscles and joints, and relieve leg pains.

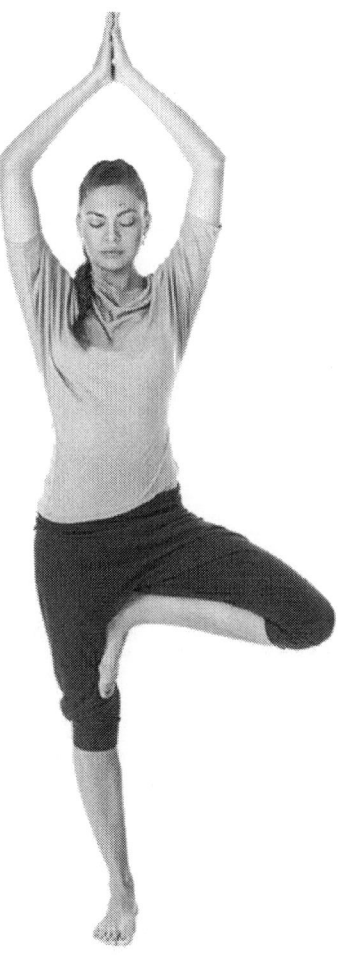

Photo Source: boston magazine.com

3. UTTANASANA OR STANDING FORWARD BEND

The Standing Forward Bend helps relieve stress, strengthen the legs, improve digestion, reduce fatigue, relieve menopause discomforts, and relieve insomnia and headache.

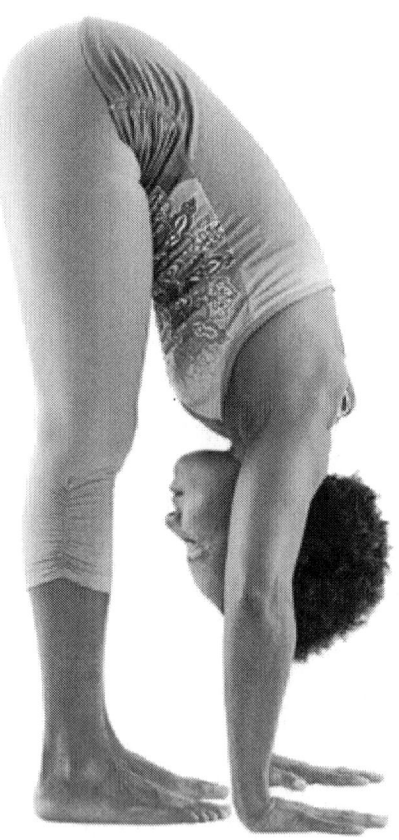

Photo Source: yogajournal.com

4. TRIKONASANA OR TRIANGLE POSE

The Triangle Pose helps relieve stress, stimulate abdominal organs, stretch abdominal and leg muscles, relieve menopause discomforts, and strengthen legs.

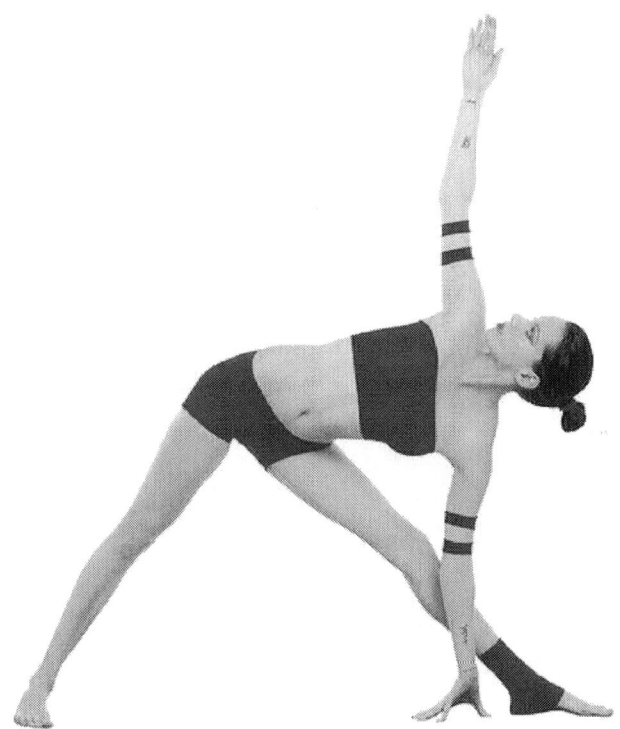

Photo Source: Wikipedia.org

5. PARIVRTTA TRIKONASANA OR REVOLVED TRIANGLE POSE

The Revolved Triangle Pose helps improve breathing by opening the chest, stretch the hips and backbone, strengthen the legs, and improve balance.

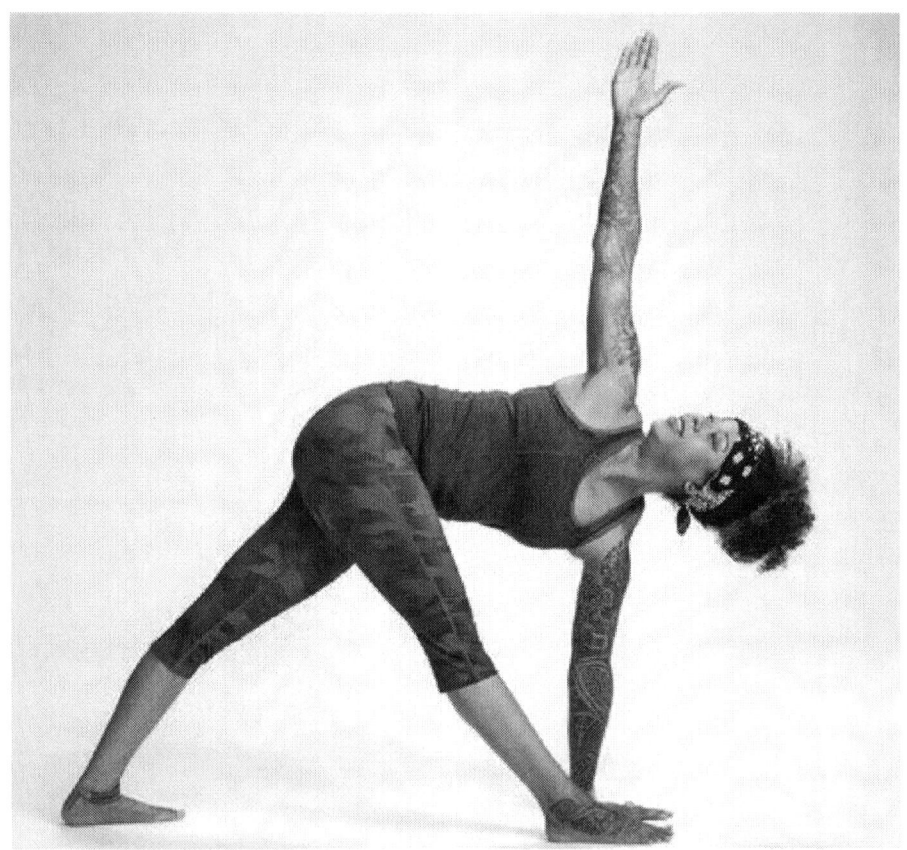

Photo Source: yogajournal.com

6. UTTHITA PARSVAKONASANA OR EXTENDED SIDE ANGLE POSE

The Extended Side Angel Pose helps strengthen the leg muscles and ankles, increase stamina, and stimulate abdominal organs.

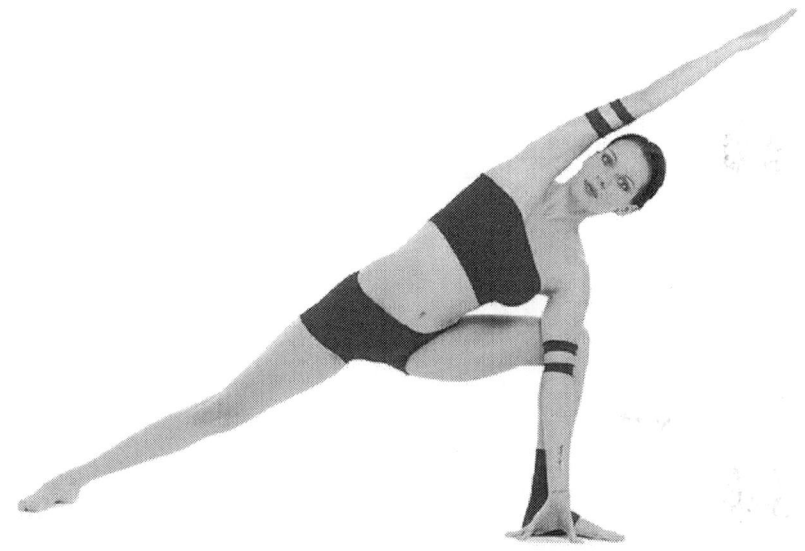

Photo Source: Wikipedia.org

7. VIRABHADRASANA 1 OR WARRIOR 1 POSE

The Warrior I Pose helps strengthen leg muscles, strengthen torso and back muscles, and stretch the chest muscles.

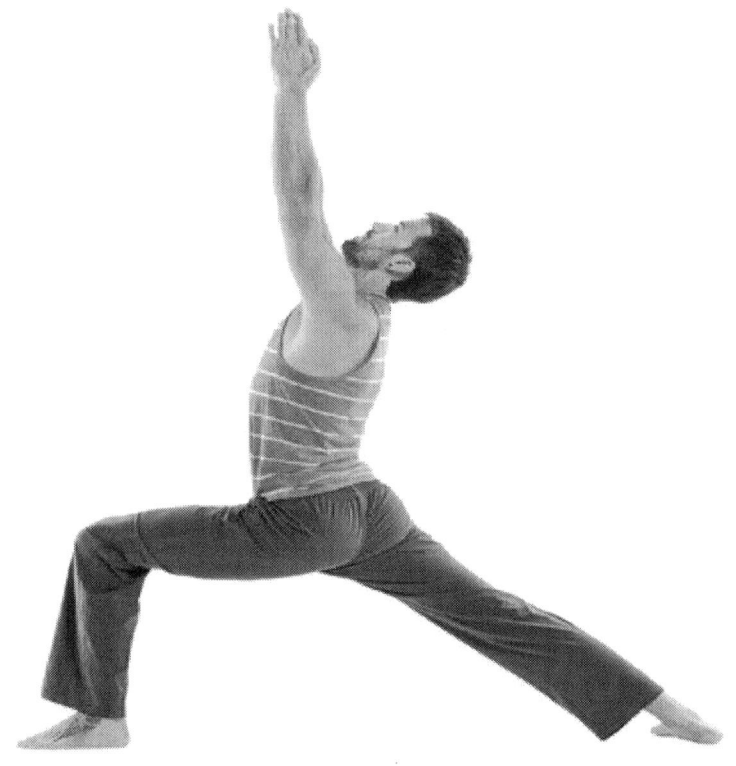

Photo Source: yogajournal.com

8. VIRABHADRASANA 2 OR WARRIOR 2 POSE

The Warrior II Pose helps increase stamina, relieve back aches, stimulate abdominal organs, and stretch leg and torso muscles.

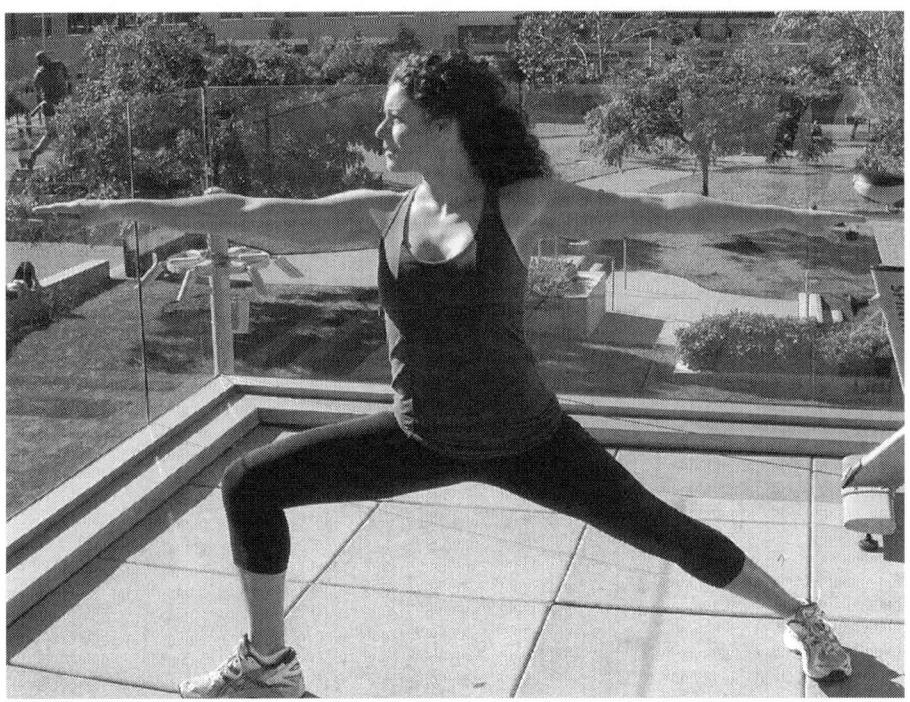

Photo Source: Wikipedia.org

17

9. VIRABHADRASANA 3 OR WARRIOR 3 POSE

The Warrior III Pose helps tone the abdominal muscles, strengthen ankles and legs, and strengthen shoulders and back muscles.

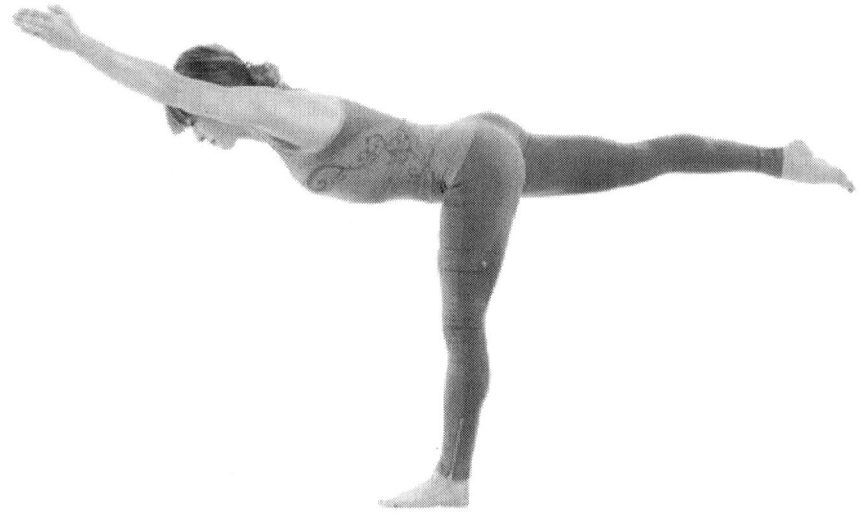

Photo Source: yogajournal.com

10. ARDHA CHANDRASANA OR HALF MOON POSE

The Half moon Pose helps strengthen the abdominal and leg muscles, improve balance and coordination, and relieve stress.

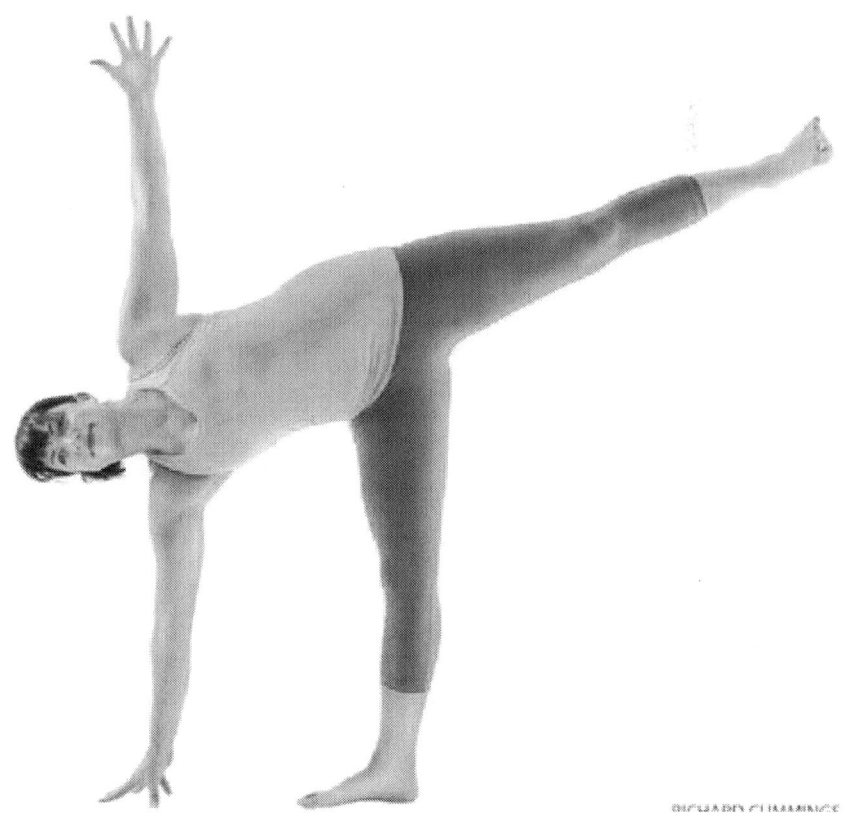

Photo Source: yogajournal.com

11. PARIVRTTA ARDHA CHANDRASANA OR THE REVERSE HALF MOON POSE

The Reverse Half Moon Pose helps strengthen the leg and lower back muscles, and strengthen the hips and shoulders.

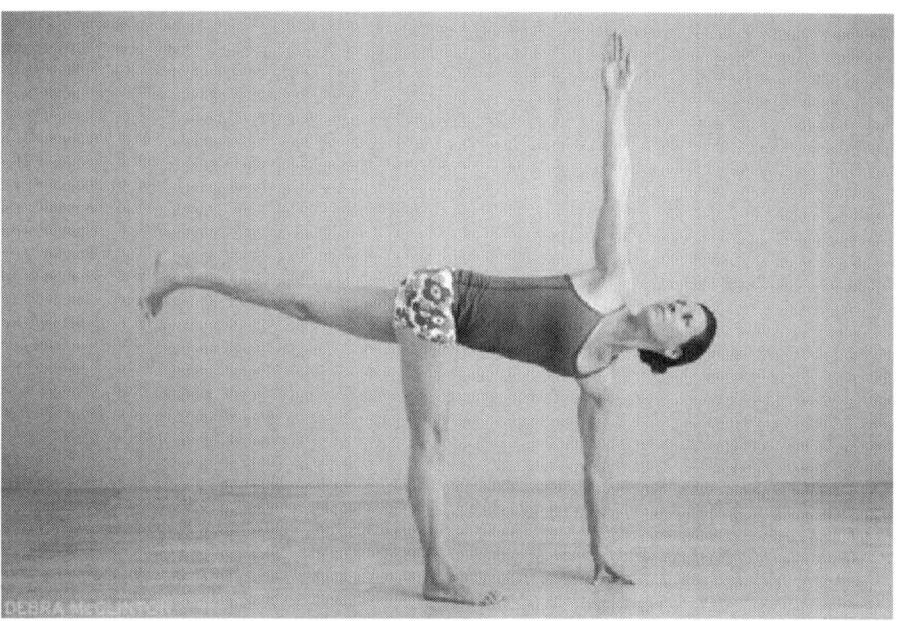

Photo Source: yogajournal.com

12. ANJANEYASANA OR THE DEEP LUNGE POSE

The Deep Lunge or Low Lunge Pose helps relieve leg pains and stretch the torso.

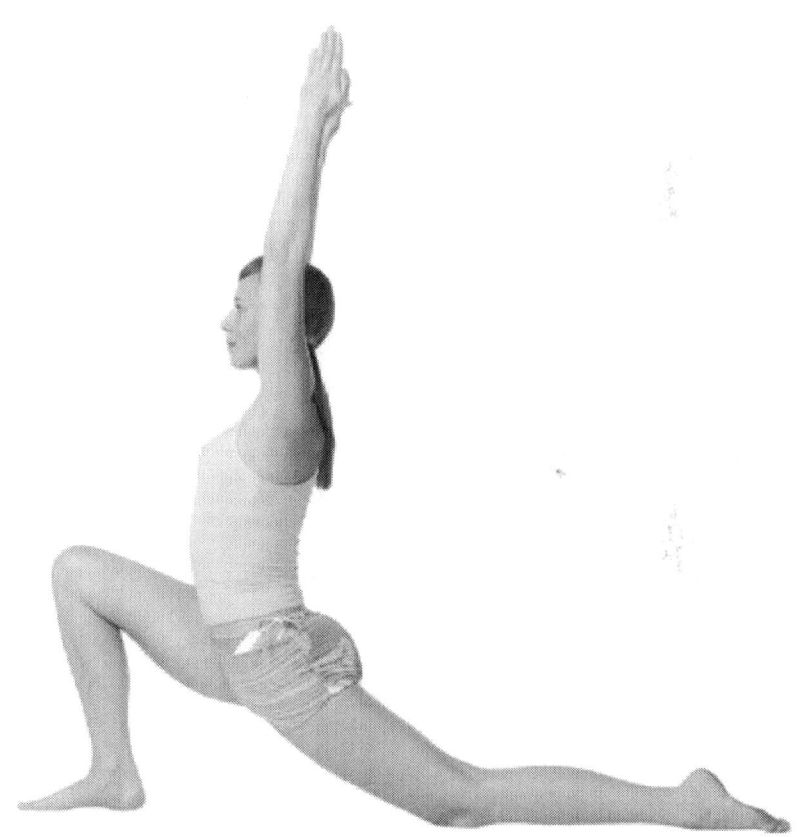

Photo Source: yogajournal.com

13. URDHVA VIRABHADRASANA II OR UPWARD WARRIOR 2

The Upward Warrior II Pose helps strengthen the leg and knee muscles, and stretch the arm and shoulder muscles.

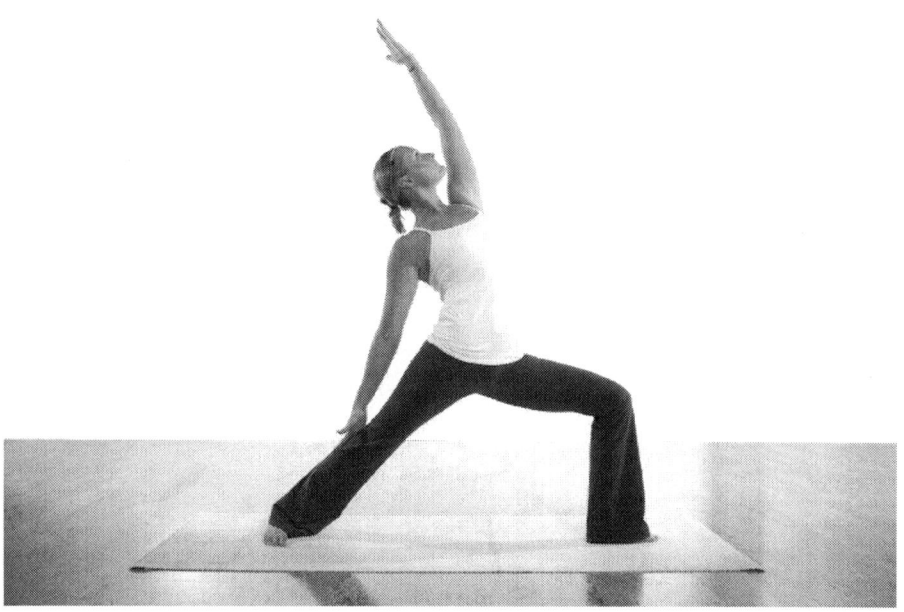

Photo Source: yogateachercentral.com

14. PARIVRTTA KONASANA OR THE REVERSE EXTENDED SIDE ANGLE

The Reverse Side Angle Pose helps stretch groin and leg muscles, increase stamina, and stimulate abdominal organs.

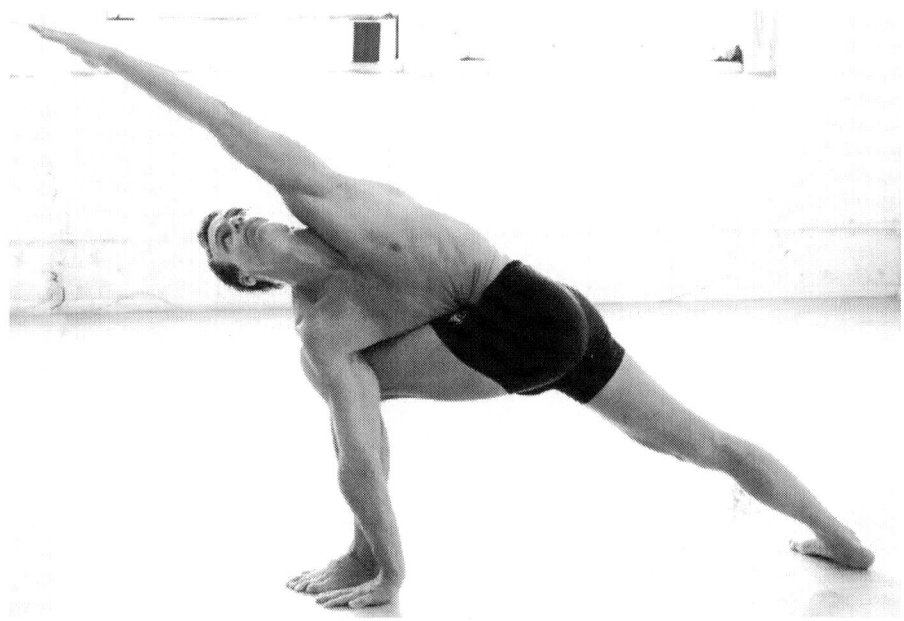

Photo Source: yogibe.tumbler.com

15. PARIVRTTA ANJANEYASANA OR REVOLVED LUNGE POSE

The Revolved Lunge Pose helps strengthen leg and hip muscles, improve digestion, relieve leg pain, and increase stamina.

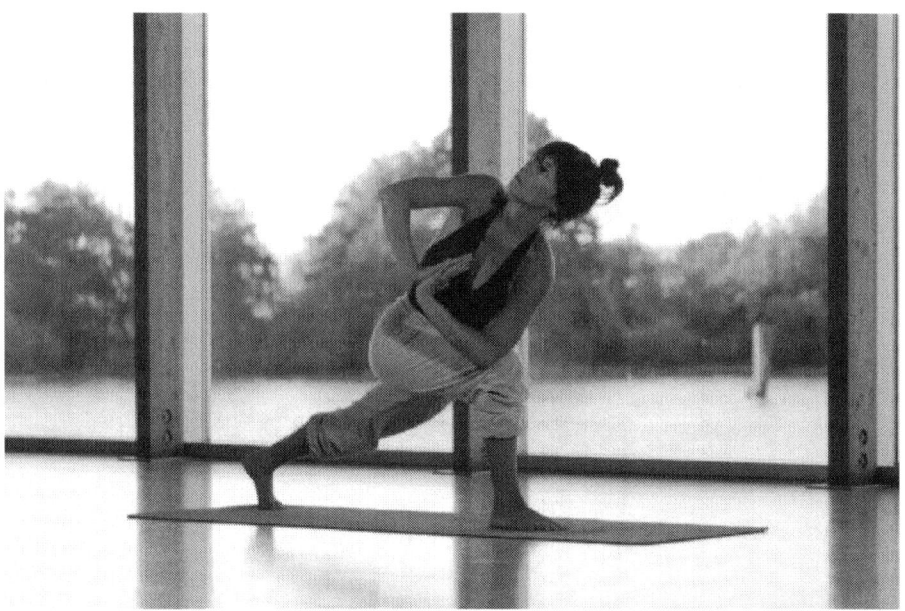

Photo Source: gaiamtv.com

16. UTKATASANA OR CHAIR POSE

The Chair Pose helps strengthen the lower back and legs, and stretch the chest and shoulders.

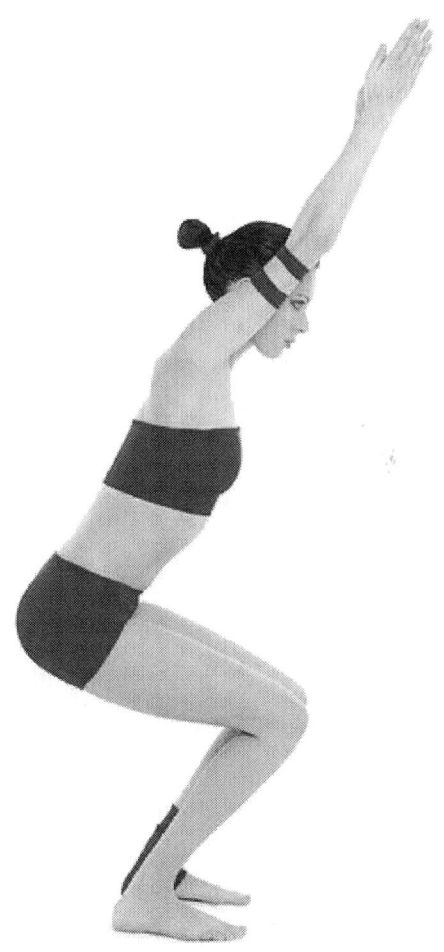

Photo Source: Wikipedia.org

17. GARUDASANA OR EAGLE POSE

The Eagle Pose helps improve balance, and stretch the legs and torso.

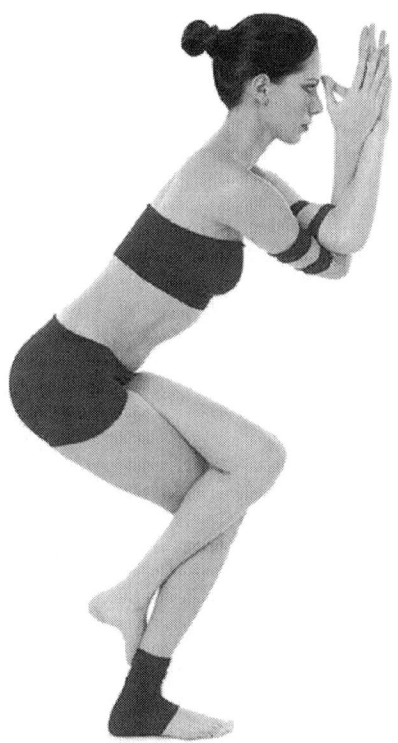

Photo Source: Wikipedia.org

18. UTTHITA HASTA PADANGUSTASANA OR EXTENDED HAND TO BIG TOE POSE

The Hand to Big Toe Pose helps improve balance and strengthen the legs and ankles.

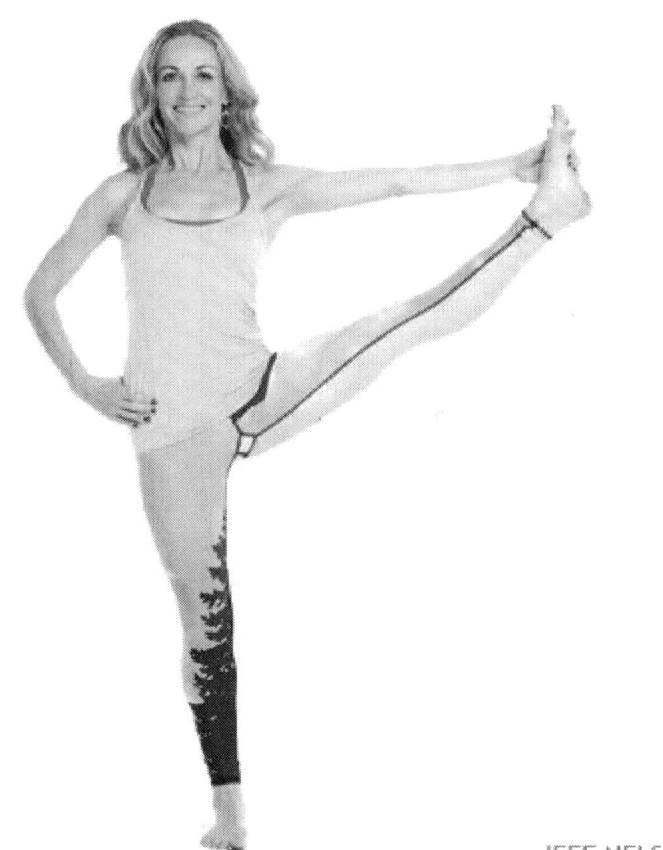

Photo Source: yogajournal.com

19. PARIGHASANA OR GATE POSE

The Gate Pose helps stretch the side of the torso and backbone, stimulate abdominal organs, and stretch the hamstrings.

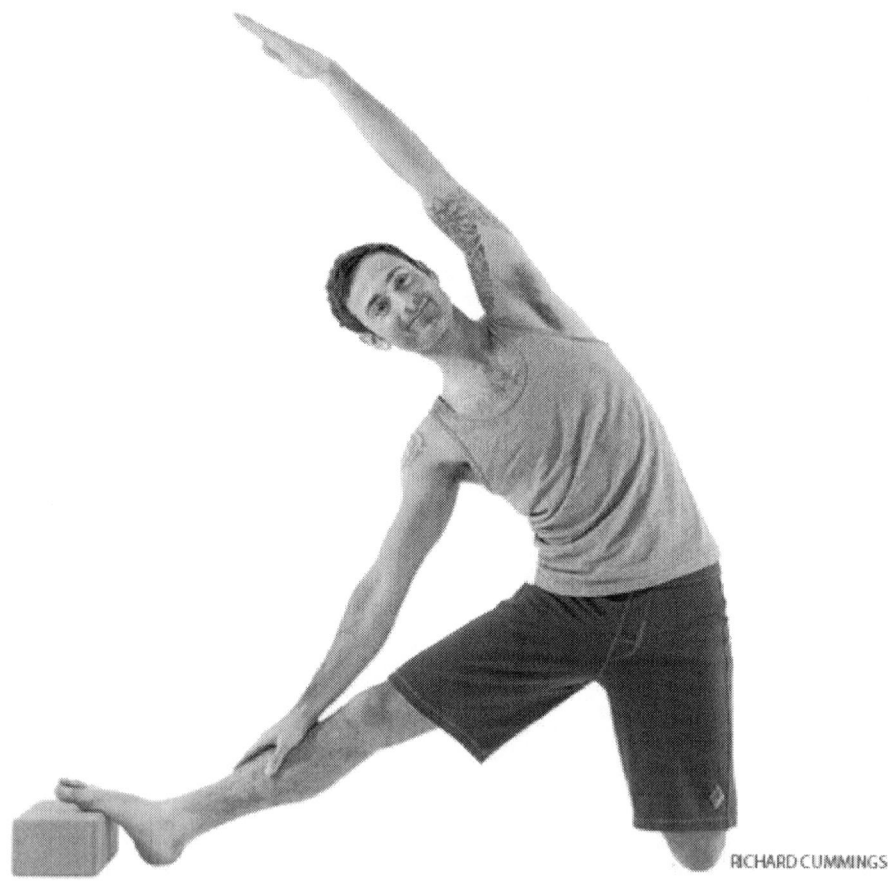

RICHARD CUMMINGS

Photo Source: yogajournal.com

20. NATARAJASANA OR LORD OF THE DANCE/KING DANCER POSE

The Lord of the Dance Pose helps improve balance, strengthen legs and ankles, and stretch leg and torso muscles.

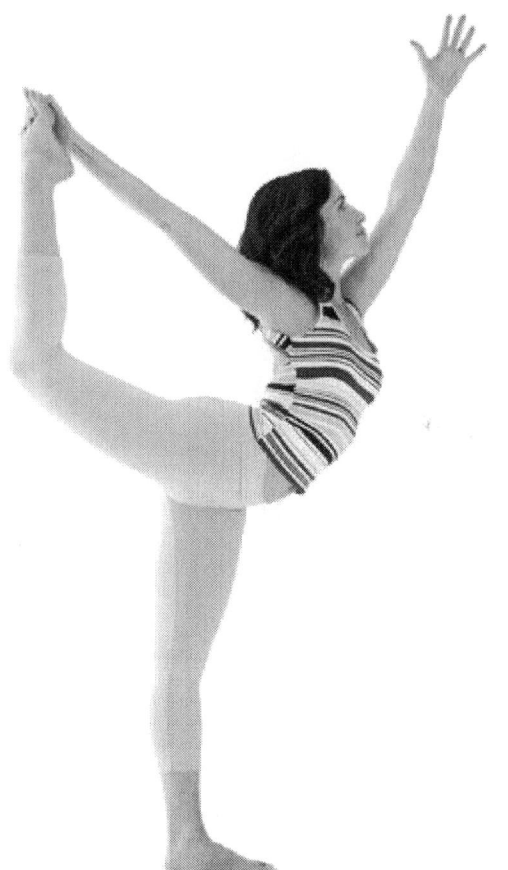

CHRIS ANDRE

Photo Source: yogajournal.com

21. PARSVOTTANASANA OR INTENSE SIDE STRETCH POSE

The Intense Side Stretch helps calm the mind, strengthen the legs, and improve posture.

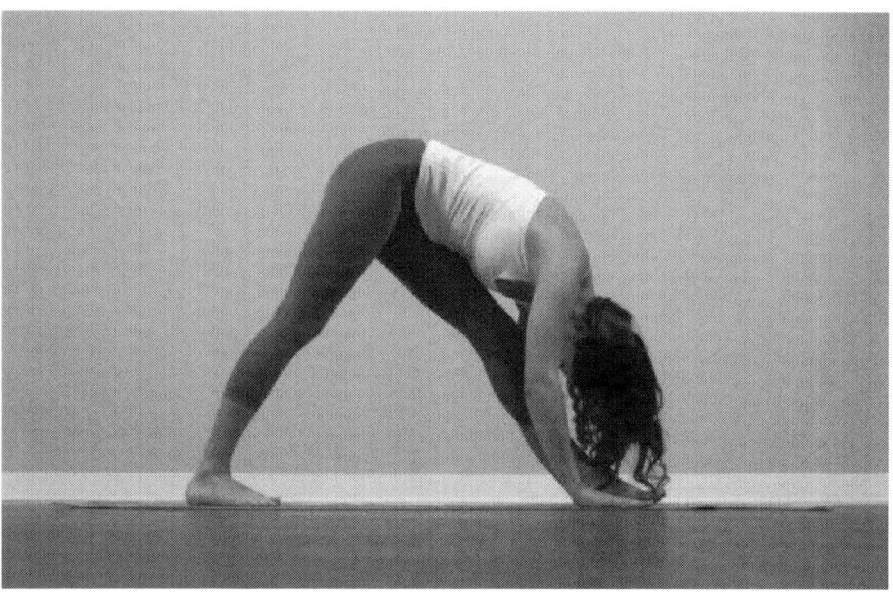

Photo Source: gaiamtv.com

22. HIGH LUNGE CRESCENT POSE

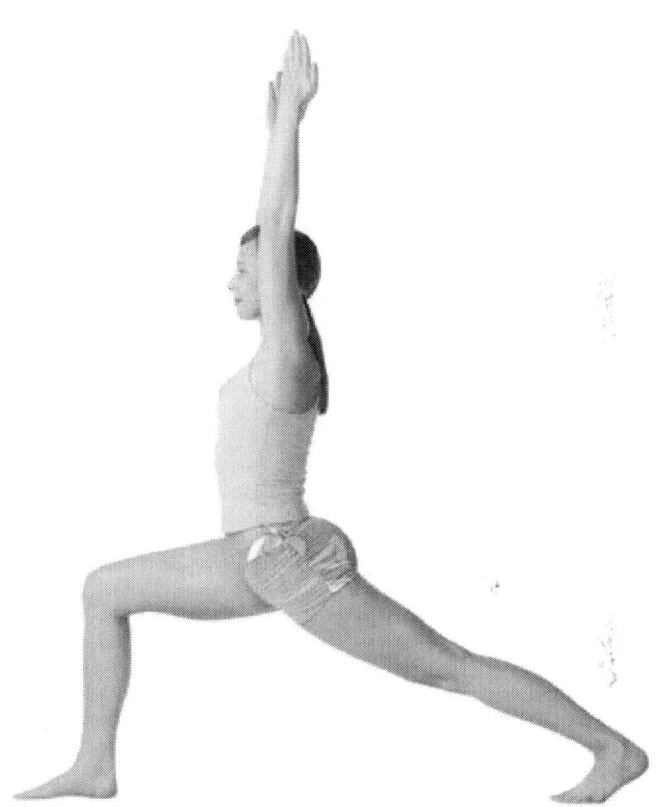

Photo Source: yogajournal.com

23. URDHVA PRASARITA EKA PADASANA OR STANDING SPLIT

The Standing Split helps calm the mind, strengthen the calves and knees, and stretch the groin and legs.

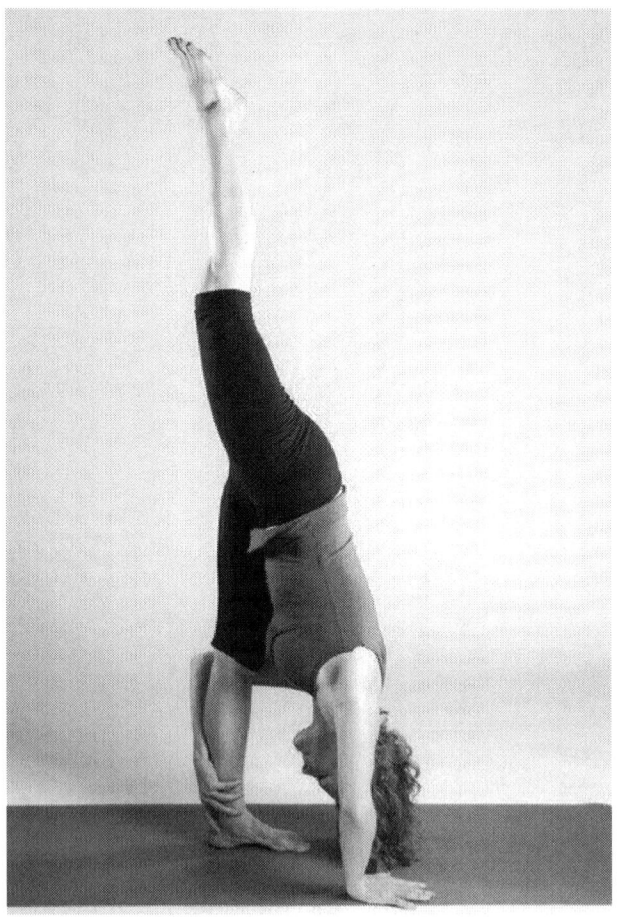

Photo Source: mantrassage.com

24. PRASARITA PADOTTANASANA OR WIDE-LEGGED FORWARD BEND

The Wide-Legged Forward Bend helps strengthen the legs and backbone, relieve back ache, and tone the abdomen.

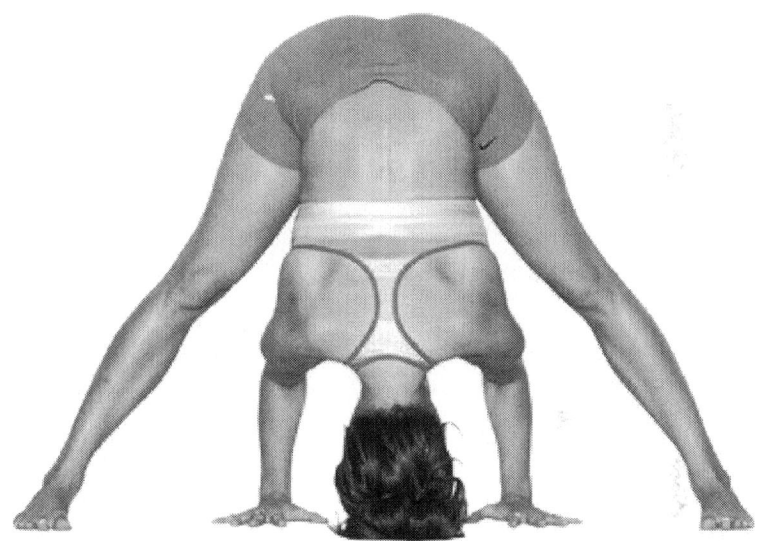

Photo Source: yogajournal.com

CHAPTER 2

SEATED POSES

Each of the different seated poses offers different and unique health benefits. Seated poses also offer a wide range of physical and emotional benefits, including the relief of anxiety, depression, and traumatic distress.

The most common seated poses that are used in many yoga classes are bound angle pose, seated twists, boat pose, lotus pose, hero, and seated forward bend. Seated poses help strengthen your spine and relax your body. These poses are great for relieving stress, strengthening and sculpting your core.

25. PADMASANA OR LOTUS POSE

Helps calm the mind, ease menstrual discomforts, stimulate pelvic organs, and stretch knees and ankles.

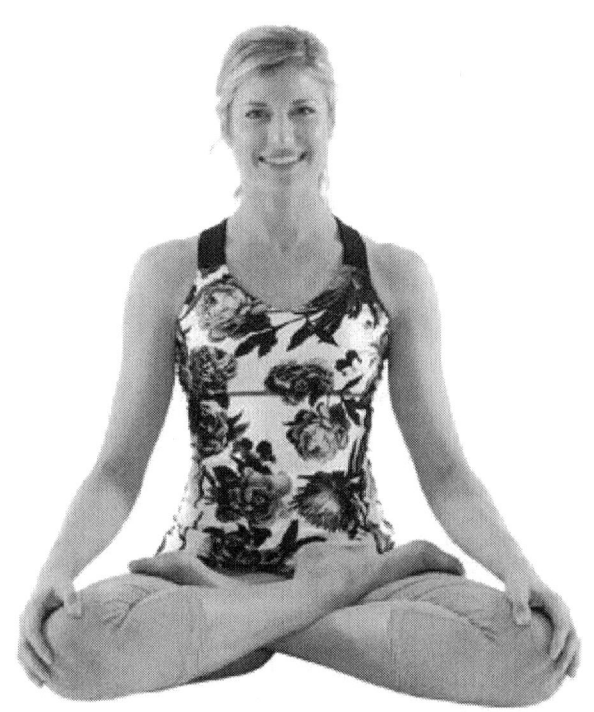

Photo Source: yogajournal.com

26 AGNISTAMBHASANA OR FIRE LOG POSE

Helps stretch the groin and hip muscles.

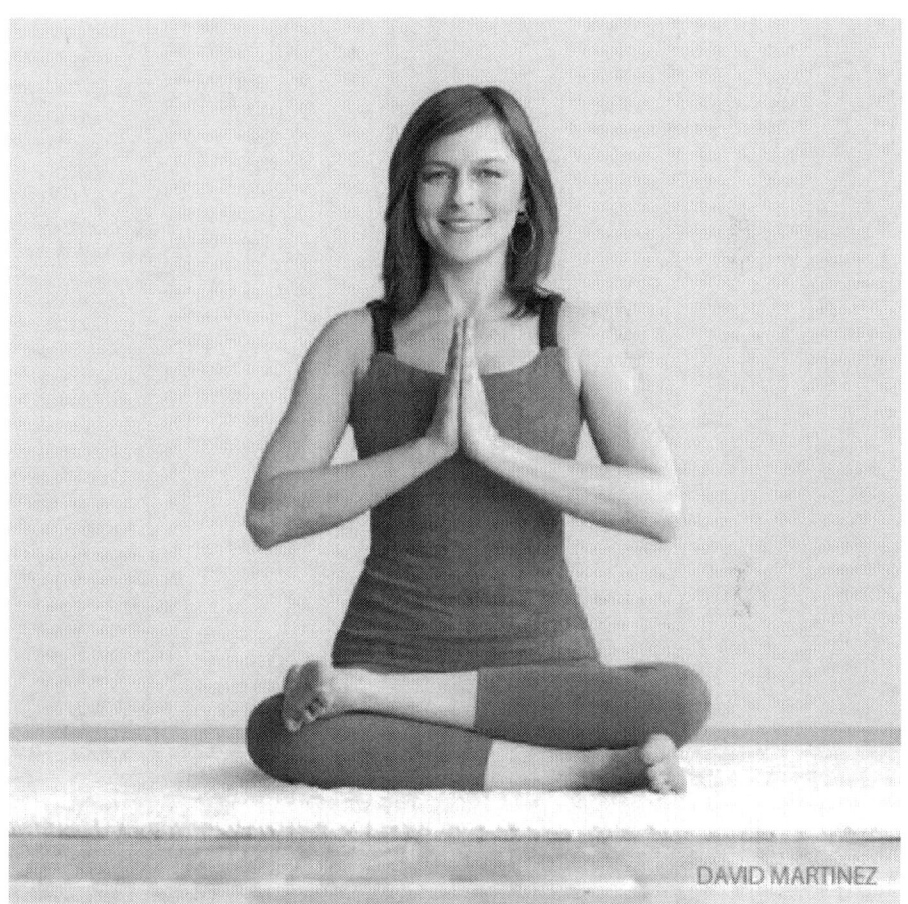

Photo Source: yogajournal.com

27. SUKHASANA OR EASY POSE

Helps stretch the ankles and knees, calm the mind, and strengthen the back.

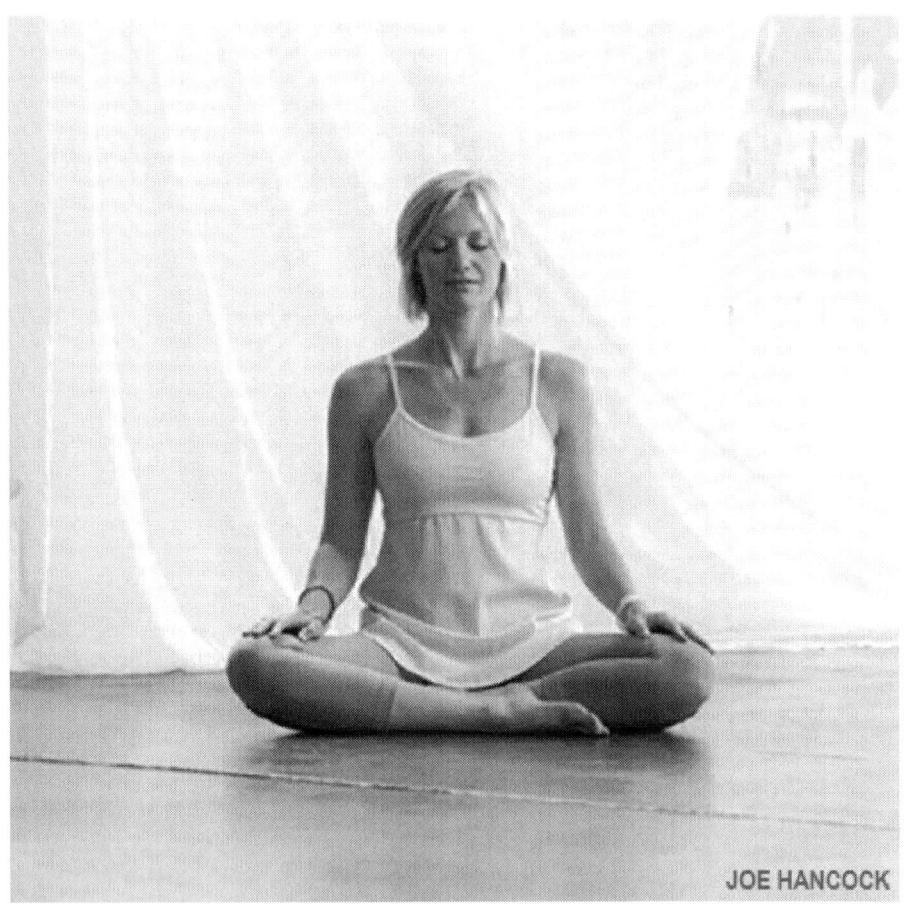

JOE HANCOCK

Photo Source: yogajournal.com

28. BADDHA KONASANA OR BOUND ANGLE POSE

Helps stretch the inner legs, ease menstrual discomforts, stimulate abdominal and pelvic organs, and improve circulation.

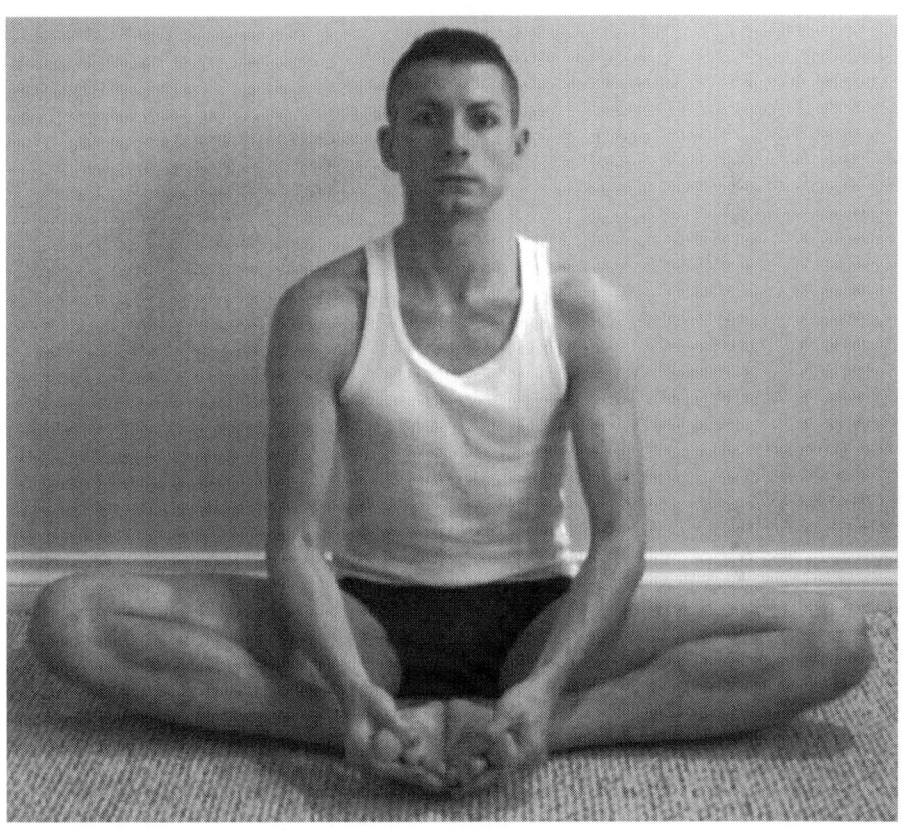

Photo Source: wikipedia.org

29. GOMUKHASANA OR COW FACE POSE

Helps stretch the leg and torso muscles.

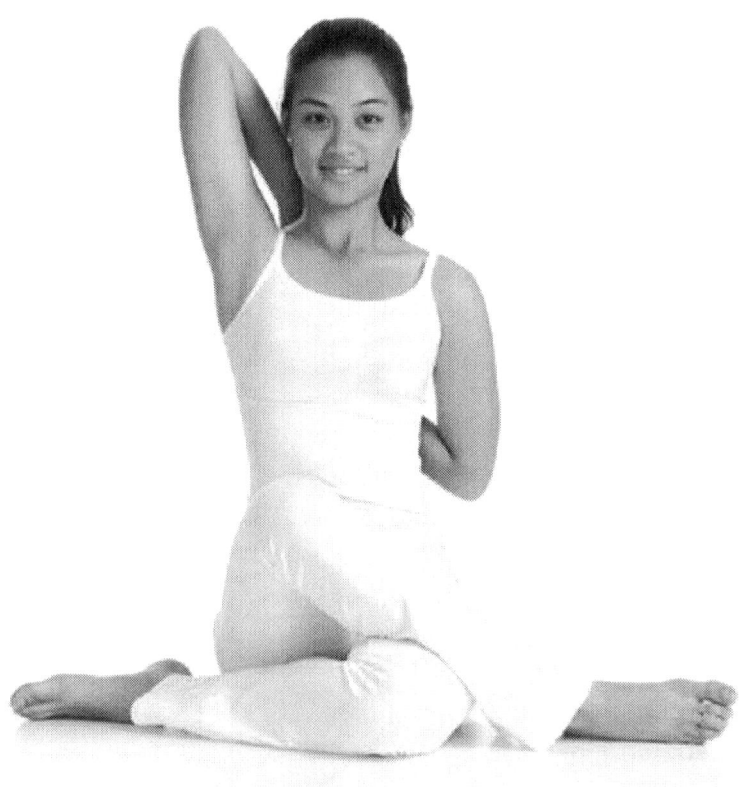

Photo Source: yogaily.com

30. ARDHA MATSYENDRASANA OR HALF LORD OF THE FISHES POSE

Helps stimulate digestion, stimulate the liver and kidneys, relieve menstrual discomforts, and stretch shoulders and hips.

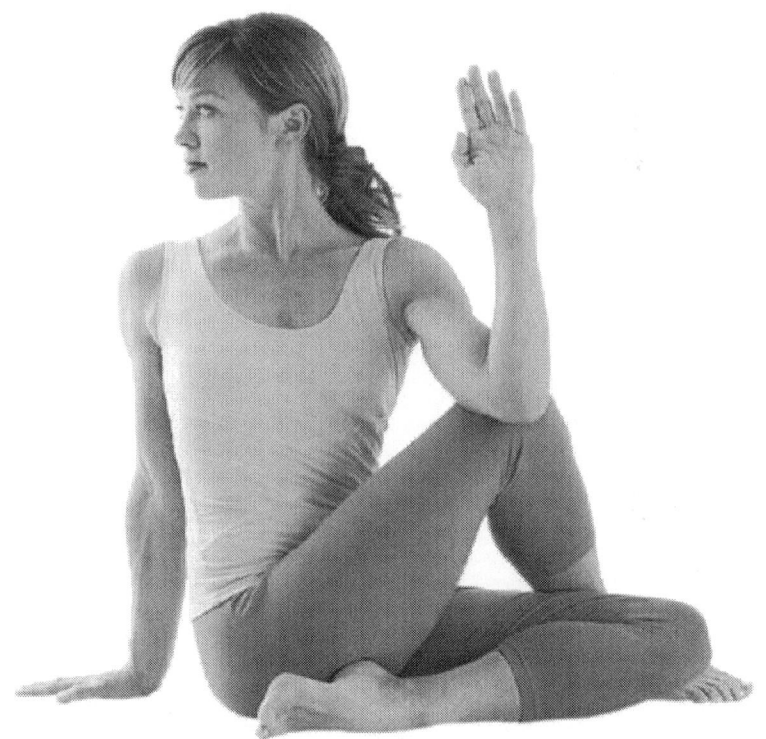

Photo Source: yogajournal.com

31. PARIPURNA NAVASANA OR BOAT POSE

Helps relieve stress, strengthen abdominal muscles, and improve digestion.

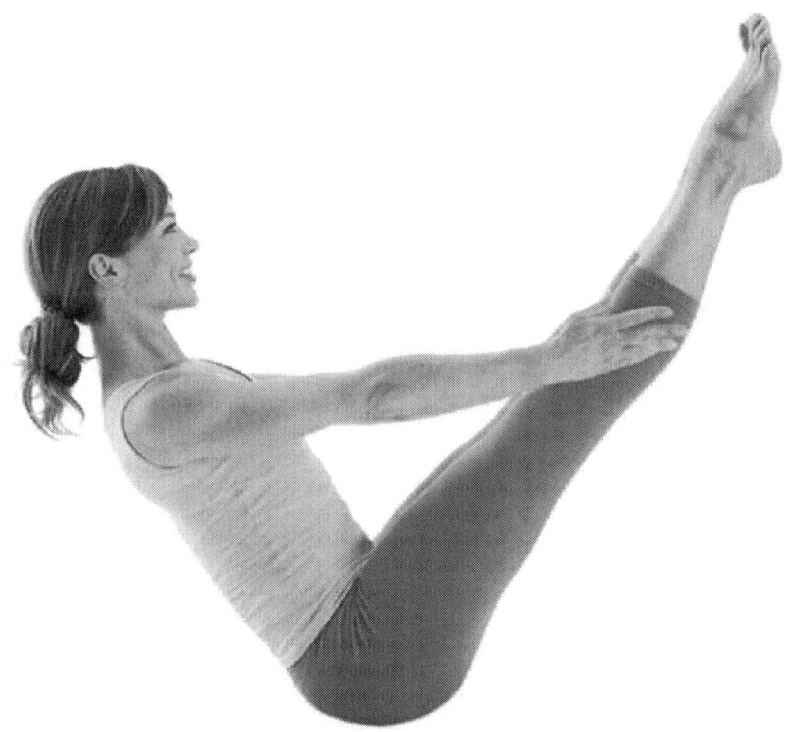

Photo Source: yogajournal.com

32. JANU SIRSASANA OR
HEAD-TO-KNEE FORWARD BEND

Helps stimulate the liver and kidneys, improve digestion, relieve stress and anxiety, ease menopause discomforts, and stretch the backbone.

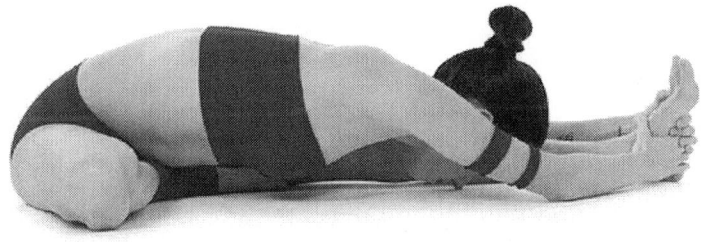

Photo Source: Wikipedia.org

33. VIRASANA OR HERO POSE

Helps stretch thighs and knees, improve digestion, relieve gas, and relieve menopause discomforts.

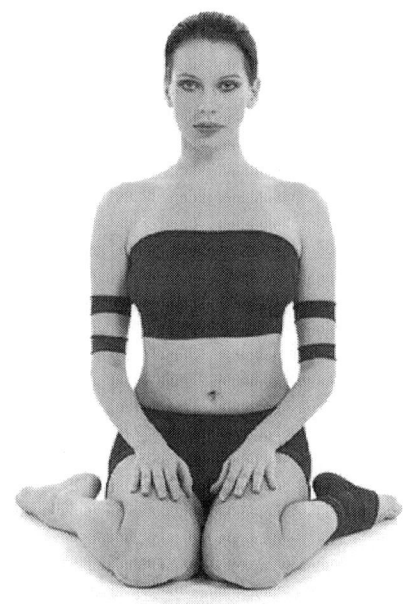

Photo Source: Wikipedia.org

34. KROUNCHASANA OR HERON POSE

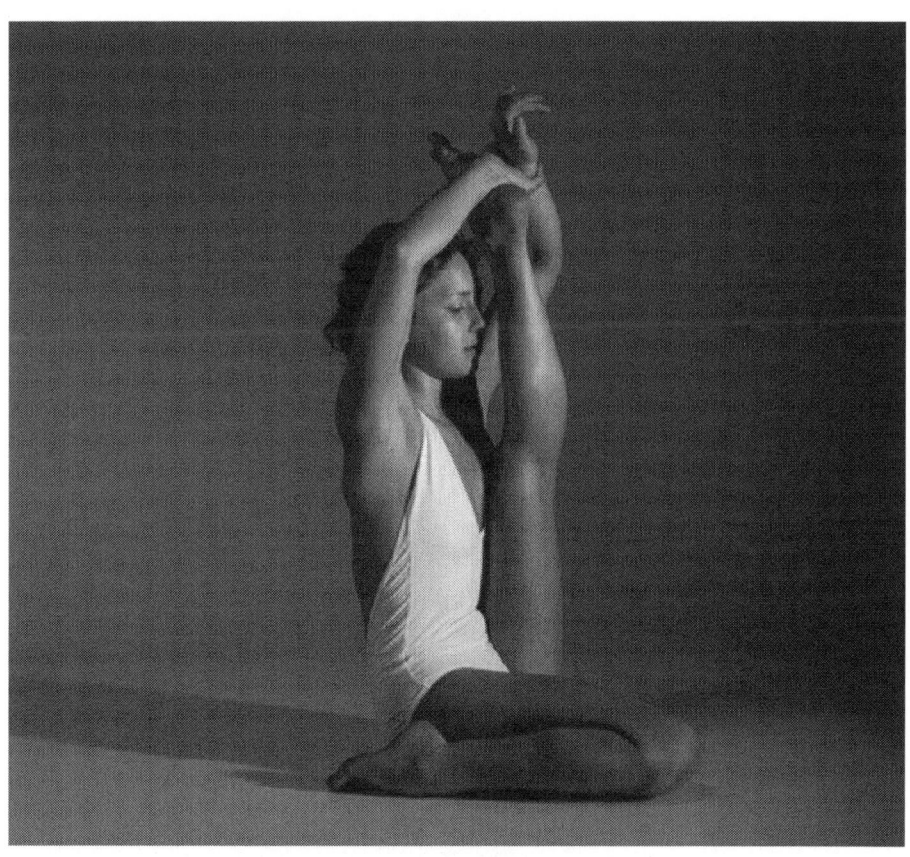

Photo Source: ashtangayoga.tumblr.com

35. MARICHYASANA III OR MARICHI'S POSE

Helps massage and stimulate the abdominal organs, relieve back ache, ease pelvic pain, and strengthen the backbone.

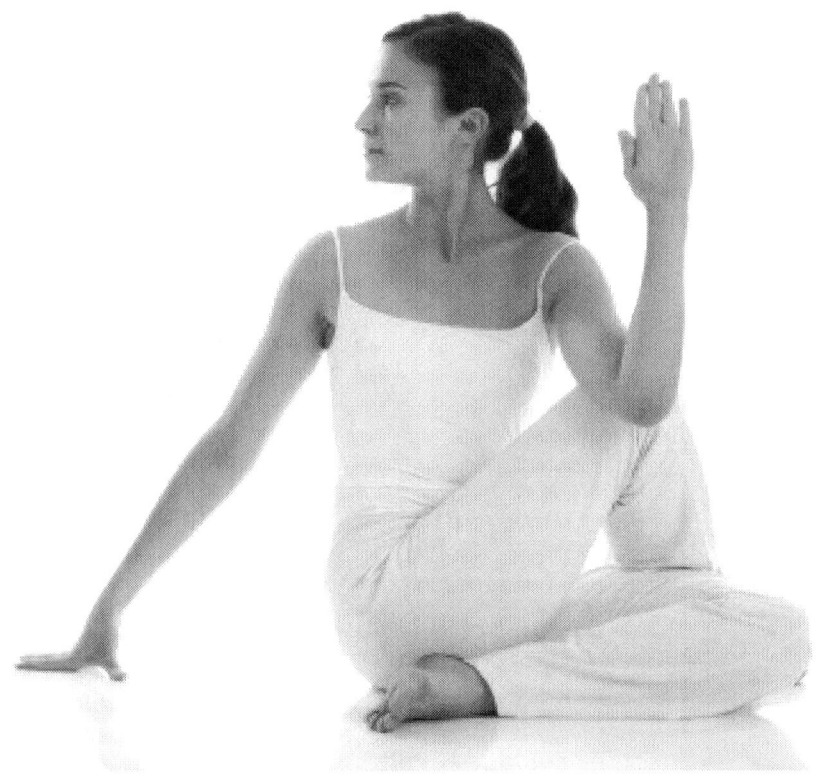

Photo Source: care2.com

36. HANUMANASANA OR MONKEY POSE

Helps stretch the leg muscles.

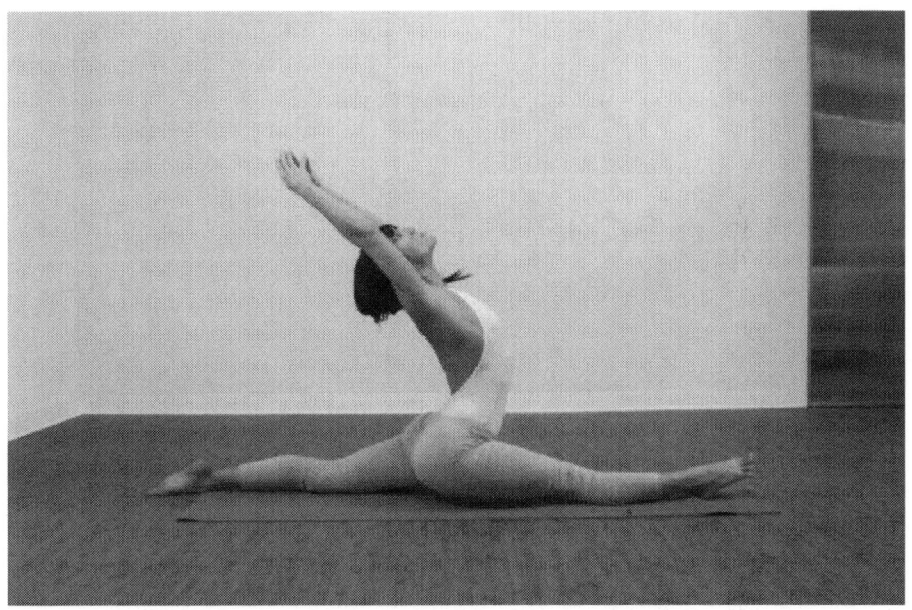

Photo Source: gaiamtv.com

37. MARICHYASANA I OR
POSE DEDICATED TO THE SAGE MARICHI I

Helps stretch the backbone and stimulate abdominal organs.

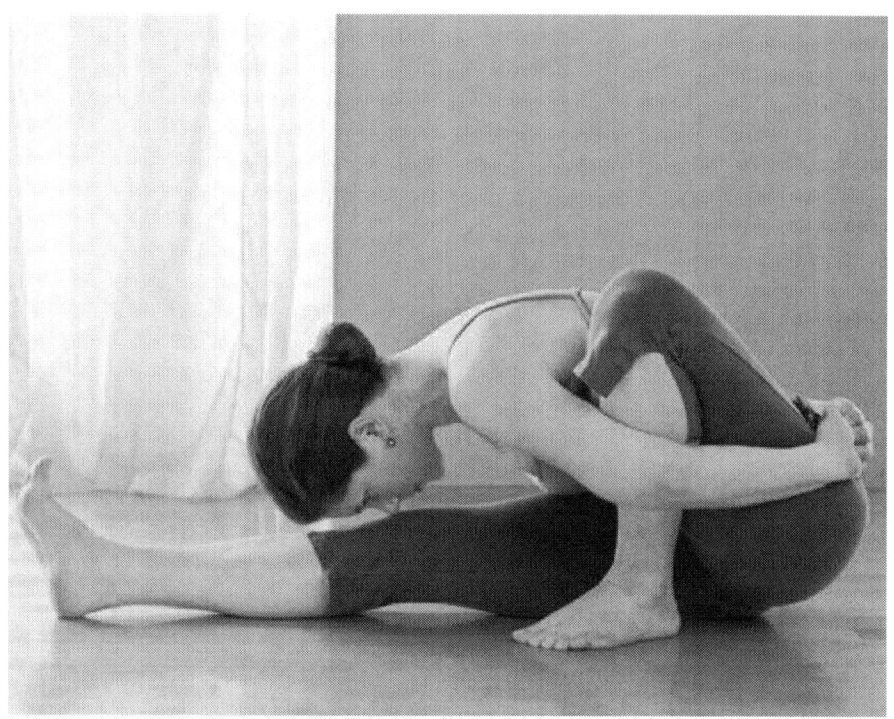

Photo Source: yogajournal.com

38. PARIVRTTA JANU SIRSASANA OR REVOLVED HEAD-TO-KNEE POSE

Helps stretch the backbone and legs, stimulate the liver and kidneys, and improve digestion.

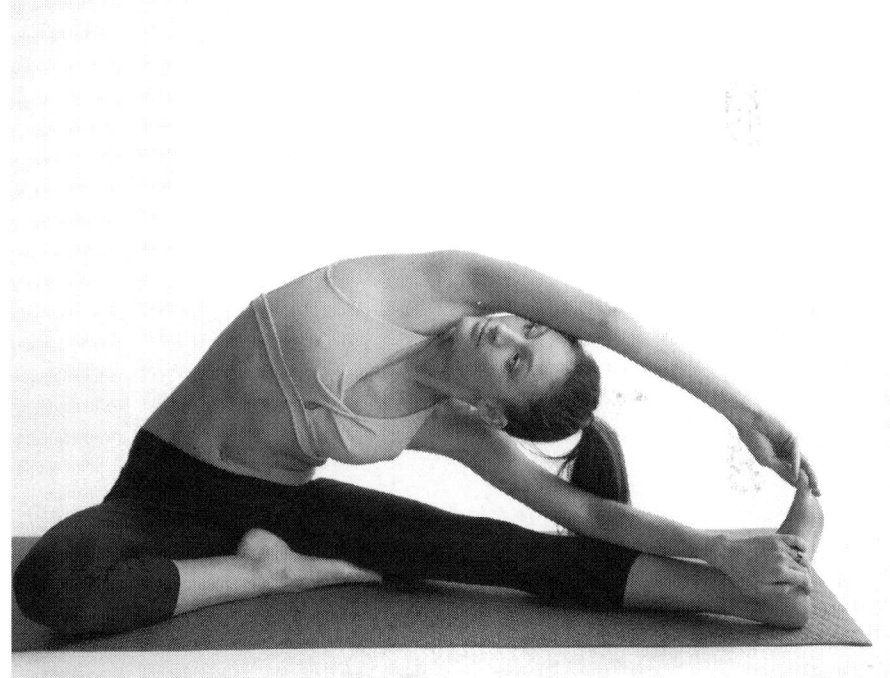

Photo Source: pixgood.com

39. DANDASANA OR STAFF POSE

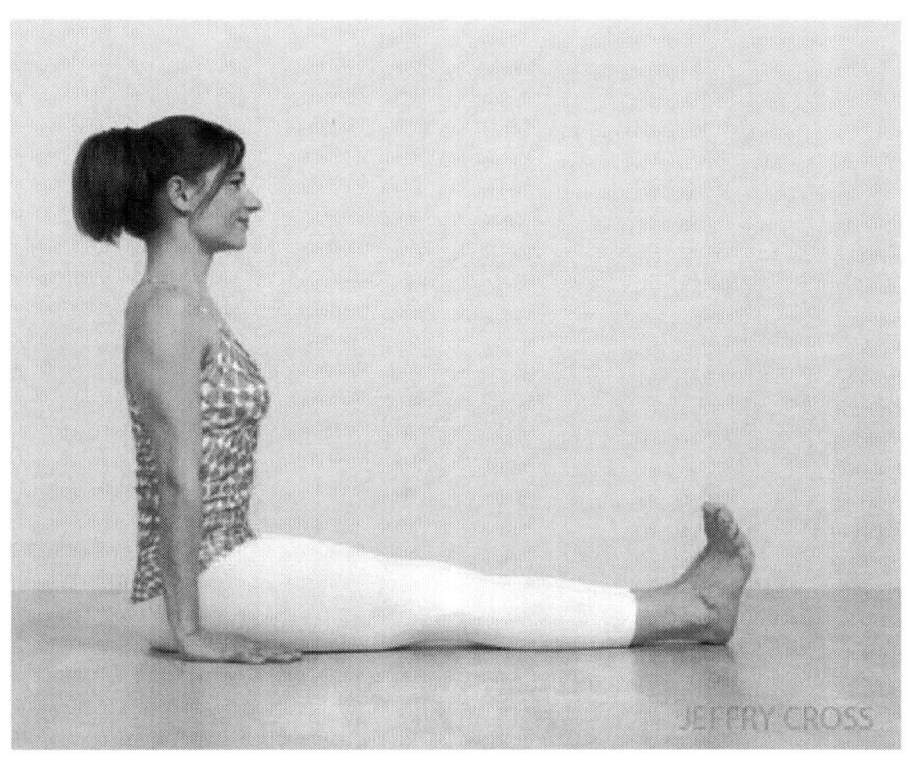

Photo Source: yogajournal.com

40. PASCHIMOTTANASANA OR SEATED FORWARD BEND

Helps stretch the shoulders and backbone, ease menstrual discomforts, stimulate abdominal and pelvic organs, and ease headaches.

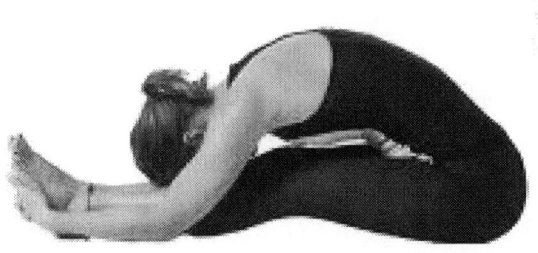

Photo Source: jadeallan.com

41. UPAVISTHA KONASANA OR
WIDE-ANGLE SEATED FORWARD BEND

Helps stimulate abdominal organs, calm the mind, and stretch the legs.

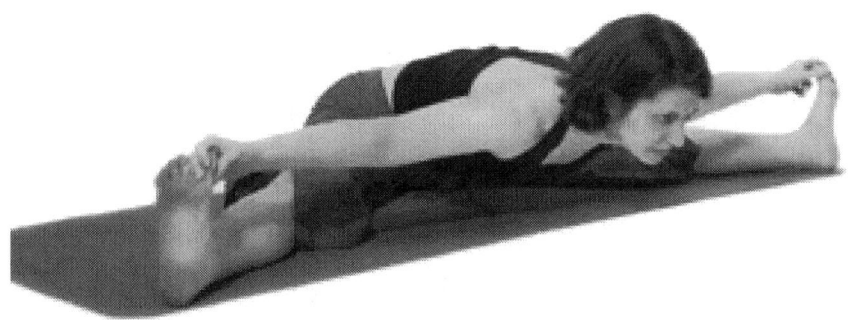

Photo Source: yogaoutlet.com

CHAPTER 3

INVERSIONS

Inversions are very challenging yoga poses that are difficult to attain for most people, but practicing these poses provides benefits that make the practice worth doing so. Inversions can give your heart a break. When you are in an upright position, the gravity pulls the fluids and the tissues in your body downwards towards your feet. If you position yourself upside down, you reverse the blood flow in your body. This will make your heart work less hard for a while.

Inversions can also improve your sense of balance and help promote better body awareness. In addition to building your core strength, these poses also force you to concentrate better and keep your focus on balancing your body.

Many experts believe that inversions can also help you maintain your youthful vitality to keep you looking and feeling young.

42. SALAMBA SIRSASANA OR SUPPORTED HEADSTAND

Helps stimulate the pituitary and pineal glands, strengthen the lungs, and strengthen the arms and backbone.

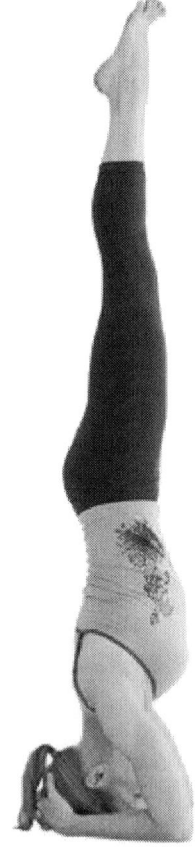

RORY EARNSHAW

Photo Source: yogajournal.com

43. SALAMBA SARVANGASANA OR SUPPORTED SHOULDERSTAND

Helps tone the legs and buttocks, improve digestion, and stimulate the thyroid and prostate glands.

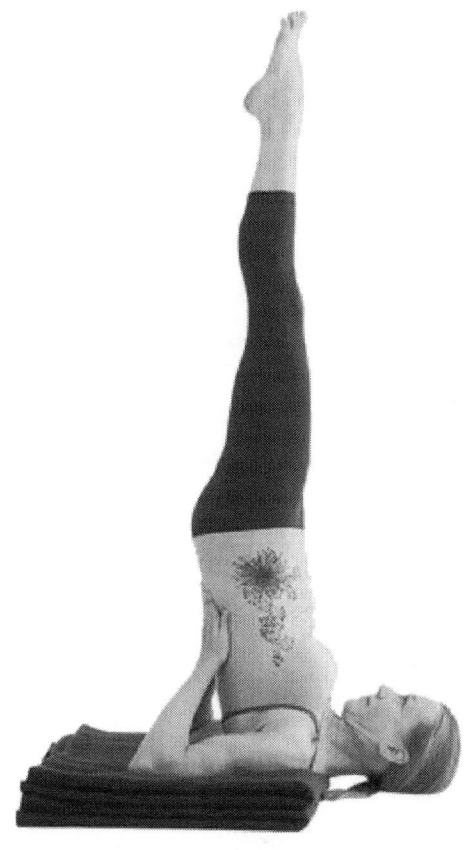

RORY EARNSHAW

Photo Source: yogajournal.com

44. PINCHA MAYURASANA OR FEATHERED PEACOCK POSE

Helps improve balance and strengthens the shoulders and back.

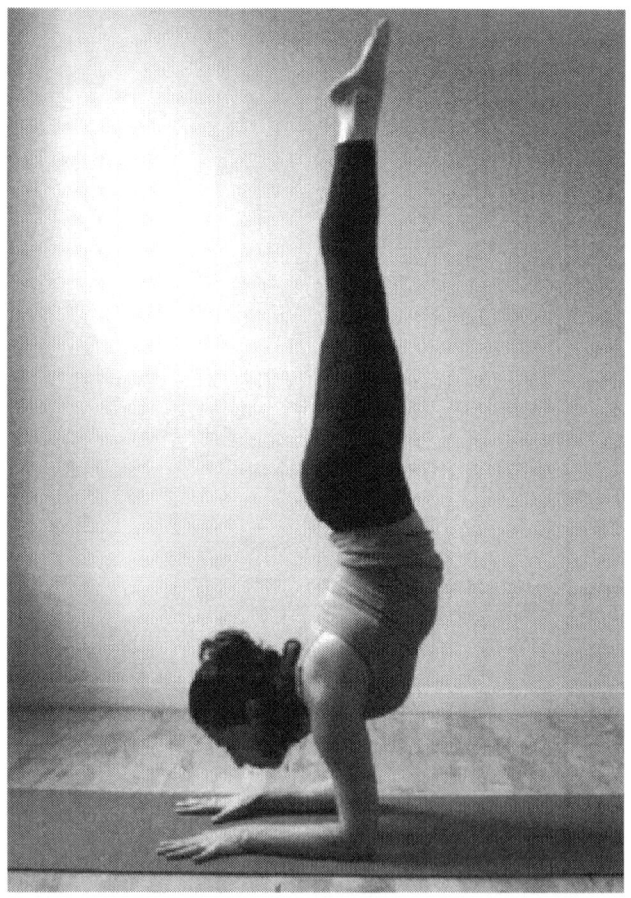

Photo Source: imgarcade.com

45. ADHO MUKHA VRKSASANA OR HANDSTAND

Helps strengthen the shoulder and arms, improve balance, and stretch the belly.

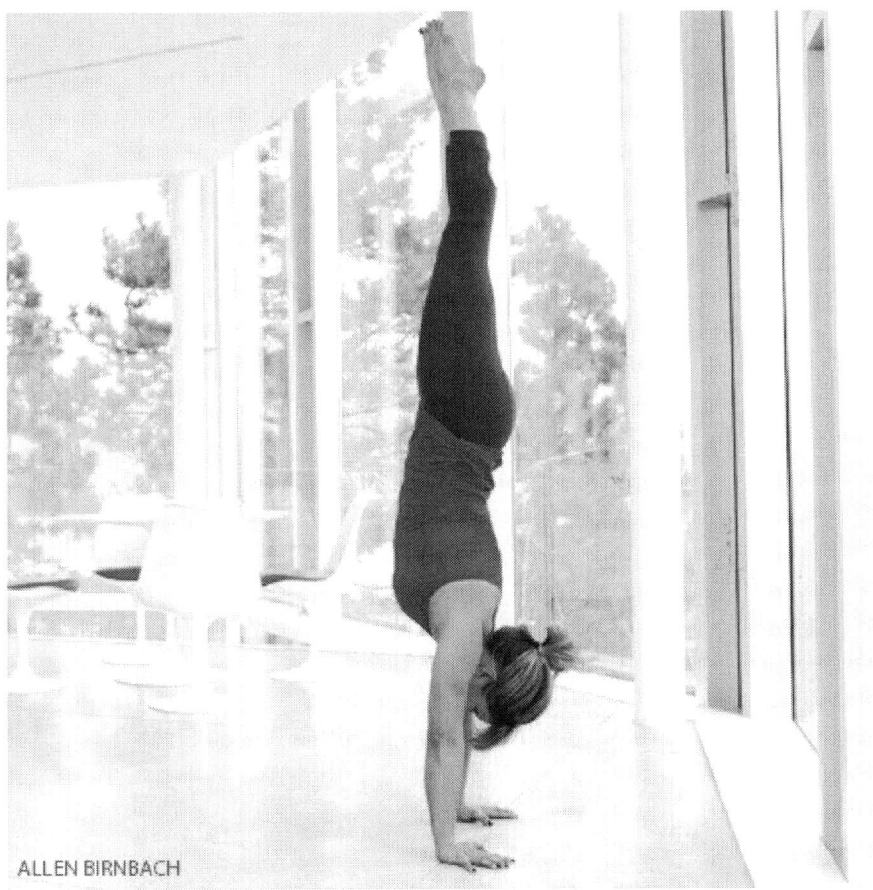

ALLEN BIRNBACH

Photo Source: yogajournal.com

46. HALASANA OR PLOW POSE

Helps stimulate abdominal organs, stretch the shoulders and backbone, and relieve menopause discomforts.

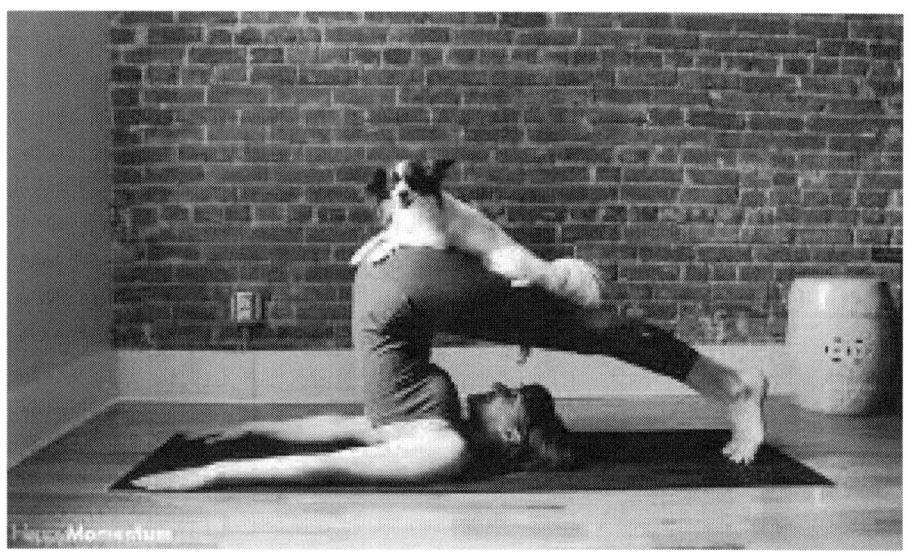

Photo Source: carenbagenski.com

47. EKA PADA SALAMBA SARVANGASANA OR ONE LEG SHOULDERSTAND

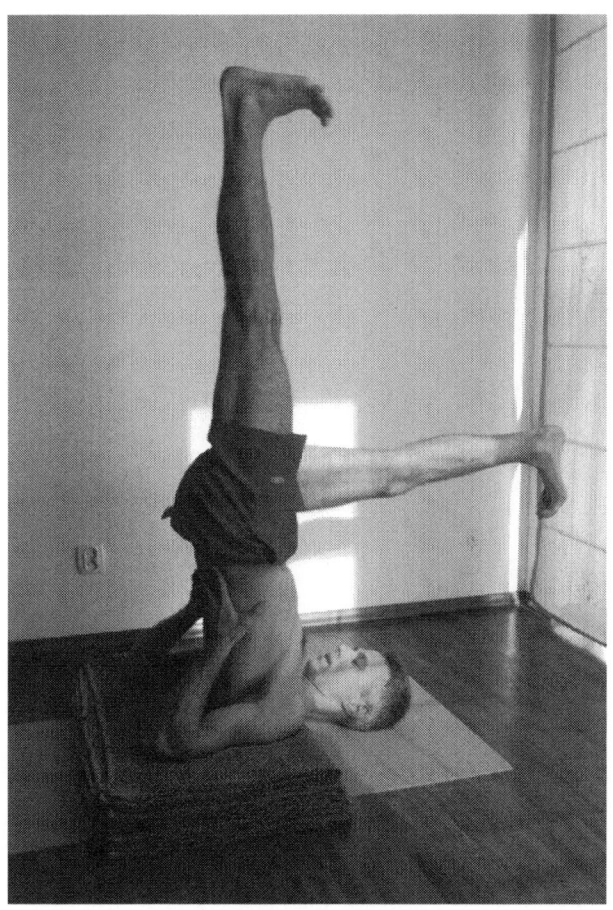

Photo Source: al-joga.pl

48. ARDHA BHEKASANA PARSVA SARVANGASANA OR HALF FROG SIDE SHOULDERSTAND

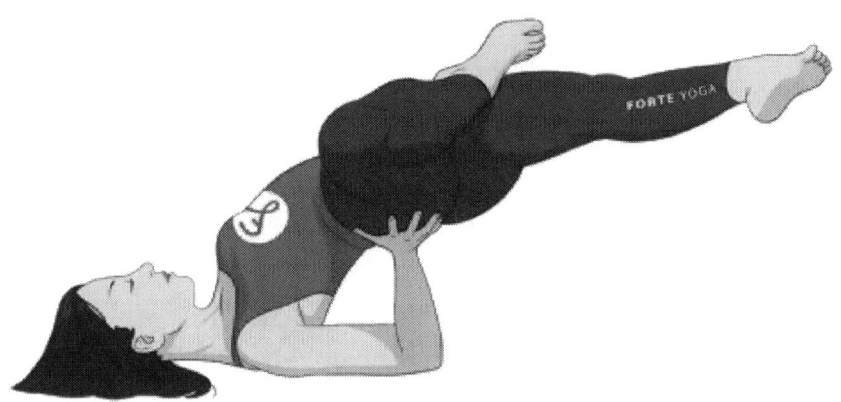

Photo Source: forteyoga.com

CHAPTER 4

ARM BALANCE

Arm balance poses help increase your strength. These also increase your body awareness and help you focus better.

These poses offer a range of health benefits. Some arm balance poses also help increase your abdominal muscle strength while most poses help flatten the abdomen. Practicing arm balance poses can be a way to minimize fear because they require you to focus on attaining and maintaining the poses by avoiding tipping over. Arm balancing is also effective in strengthening your arms and improving balance.

49. BAKASANA OR CROW POSE

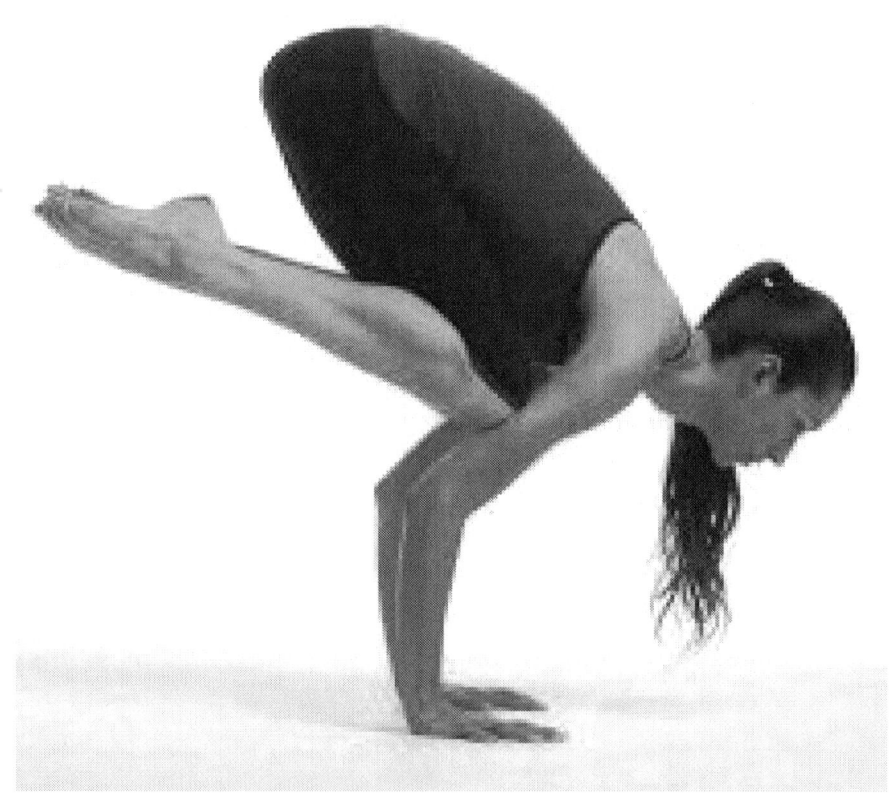

Photo Source: tarastiles.com

50. DOLPHIN PLANK POSE

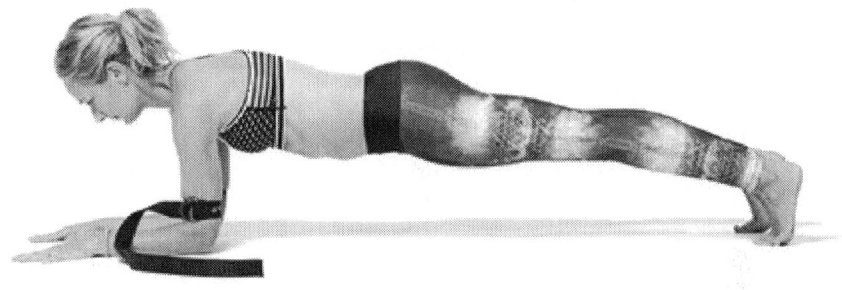

Photo Source: yogajournal.com

51. MAYURASANA OR PEACOCK POSE

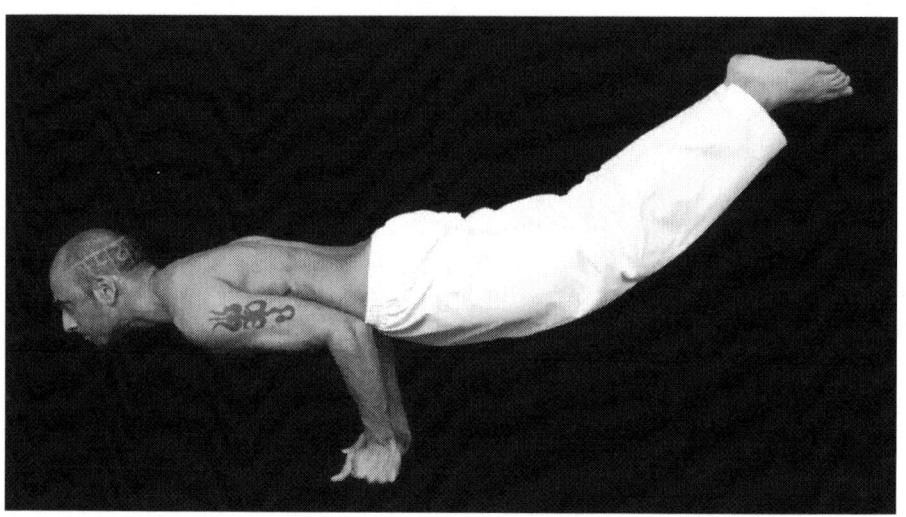

Photo Source: chikri.com

52. ONE ARM PEACOCK POSE

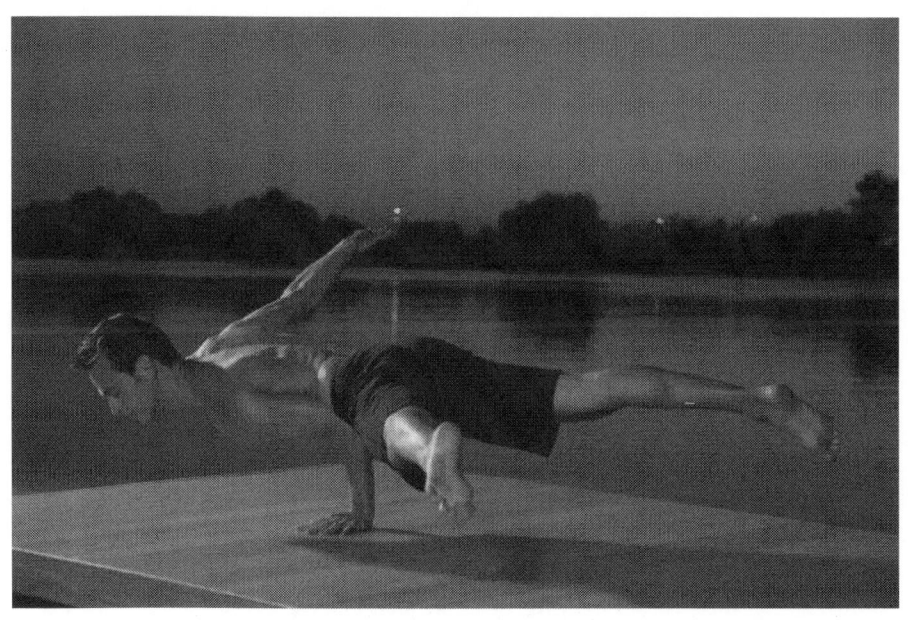

Photo Source: vegacommunity.com

53. ASTAVAKRASANA OR EIGHT-ANGLE POSE

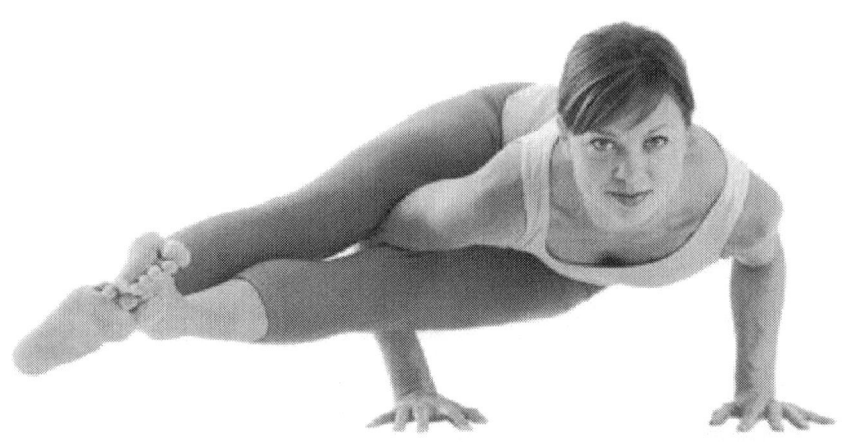

Photo Source: yogajournal.com

54. CHATURANGA DANDASANA OR FOUR-LIMBED STAFF POSE

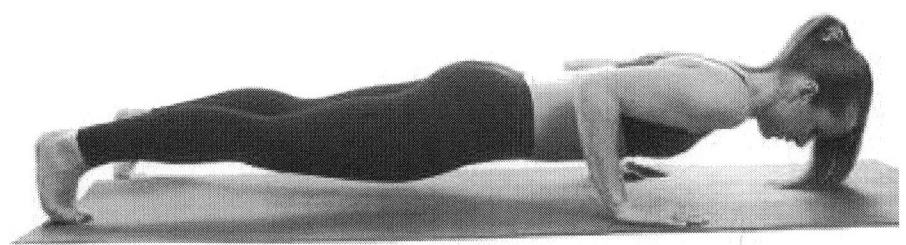

Photo Source: tummee.com

55. FIREFLY POSE

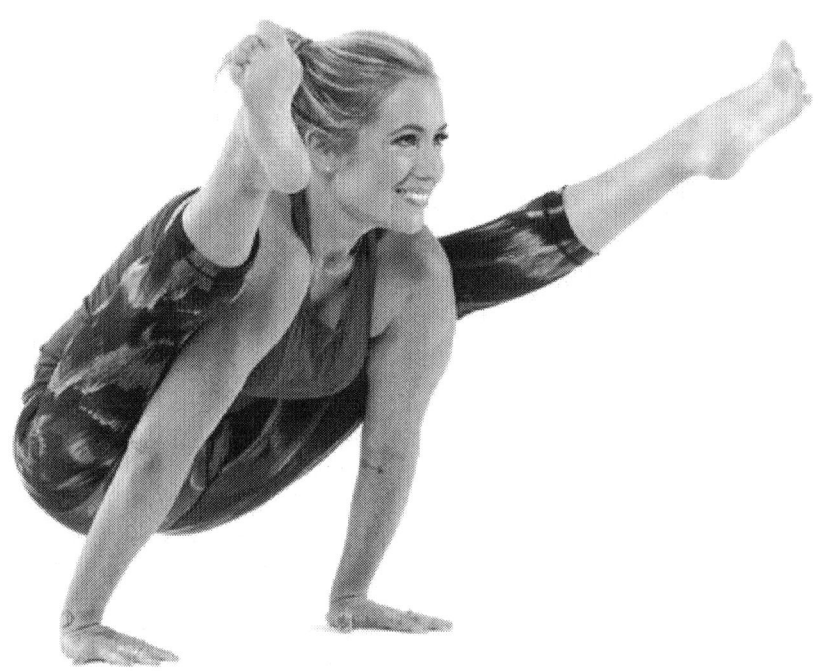

Photo Source: yogajournal.com

56. PLANK POSE

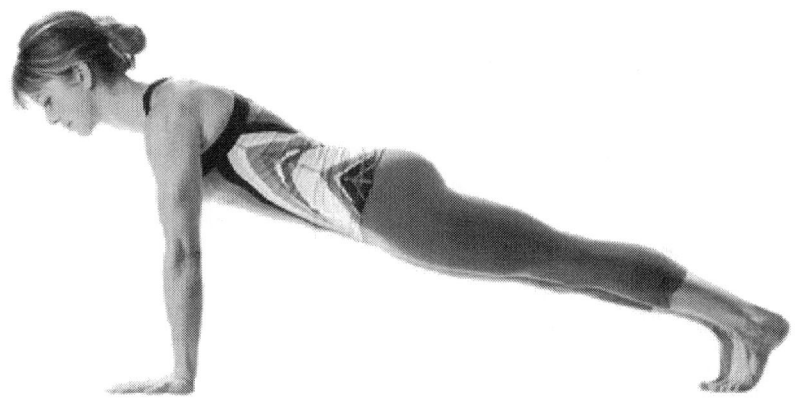

Photo Source: yogajournal.com

57. EKA PADA KOUNDINYANASANA I OR POSE DEDICATED TO THE SAGE KOUNDINYA I

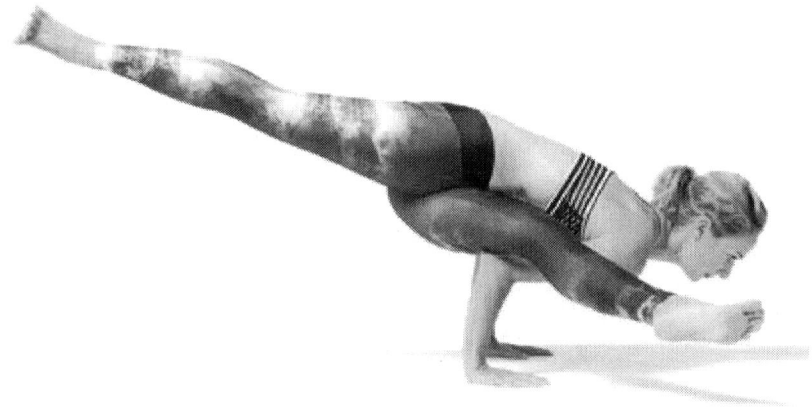

Photo Source: yogajournal.com

58. EKA PADA GALAVASANA OR FLYING CROW/PIGEON POSE

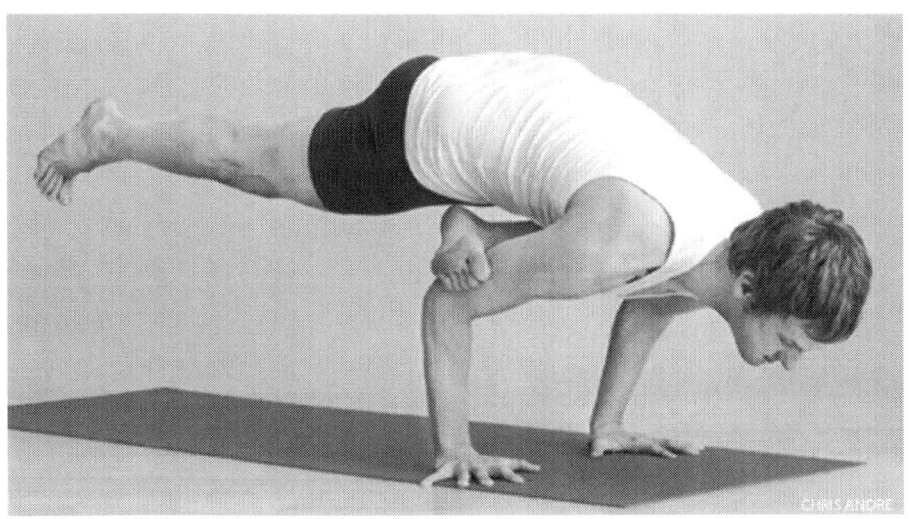

Photo Source: yogajournal.com

59. PARSVA DANDASANA OR
SIDE STAFF/PLANK POSE

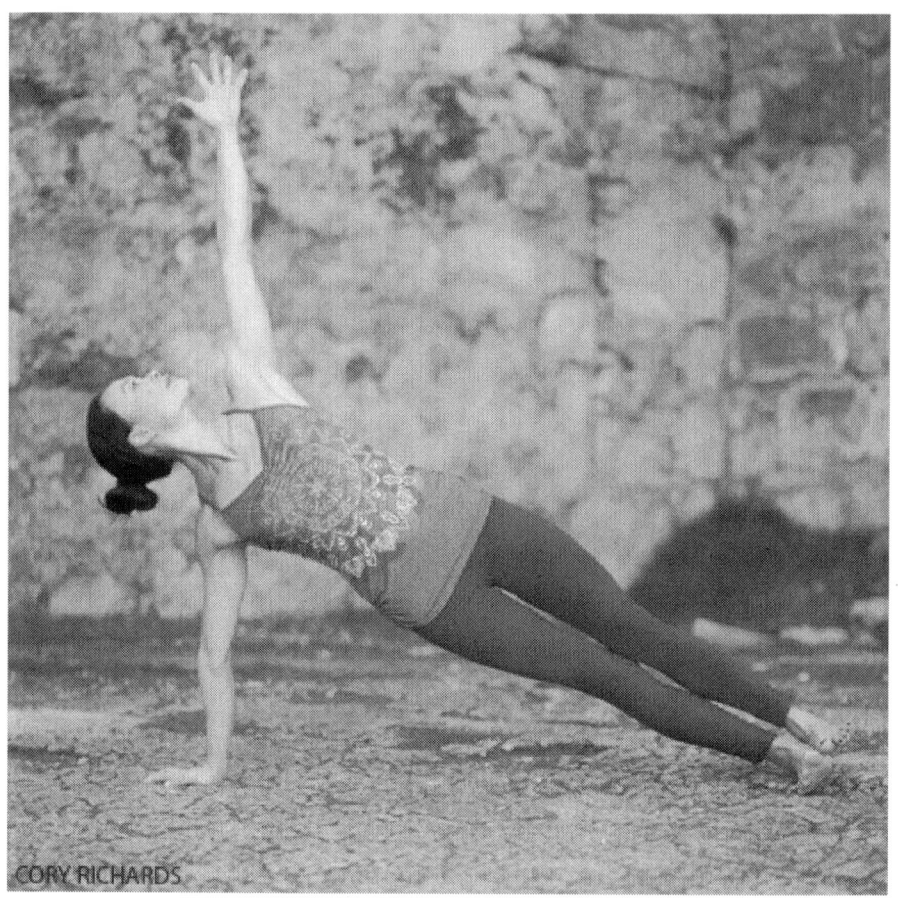

Photo Source: yogajournal.com

60. SCALE POSE OR TOLASANA

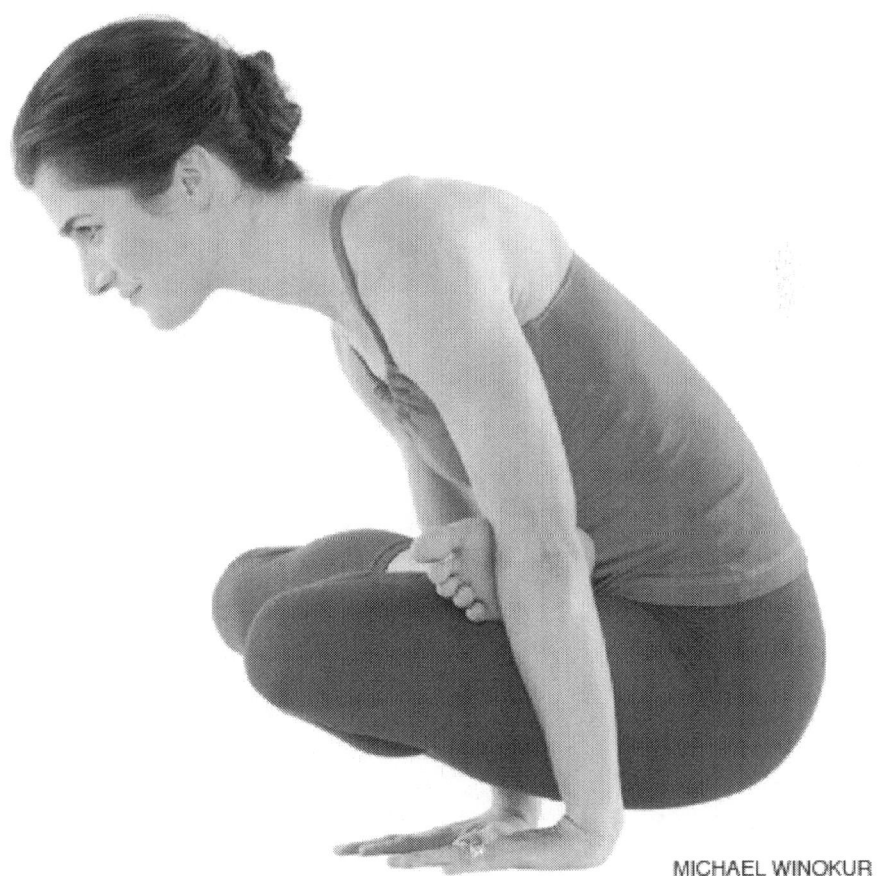

MICHAEL WINOKUR

Photo Source: yogajournal.com

61. BHUJAPIDASANA OR SHOULDER-PRESSING POSE

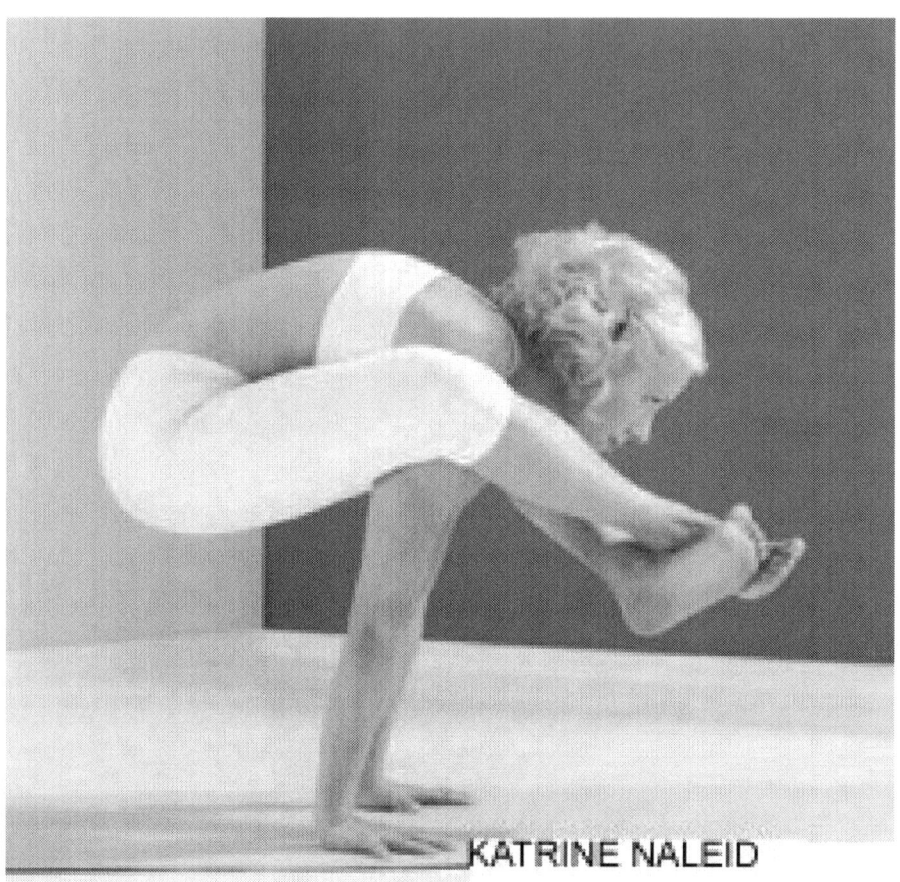

Photo Source: yogajournal.com

62. SCORPION POSE OR BHUJA VRISCHIKASANA

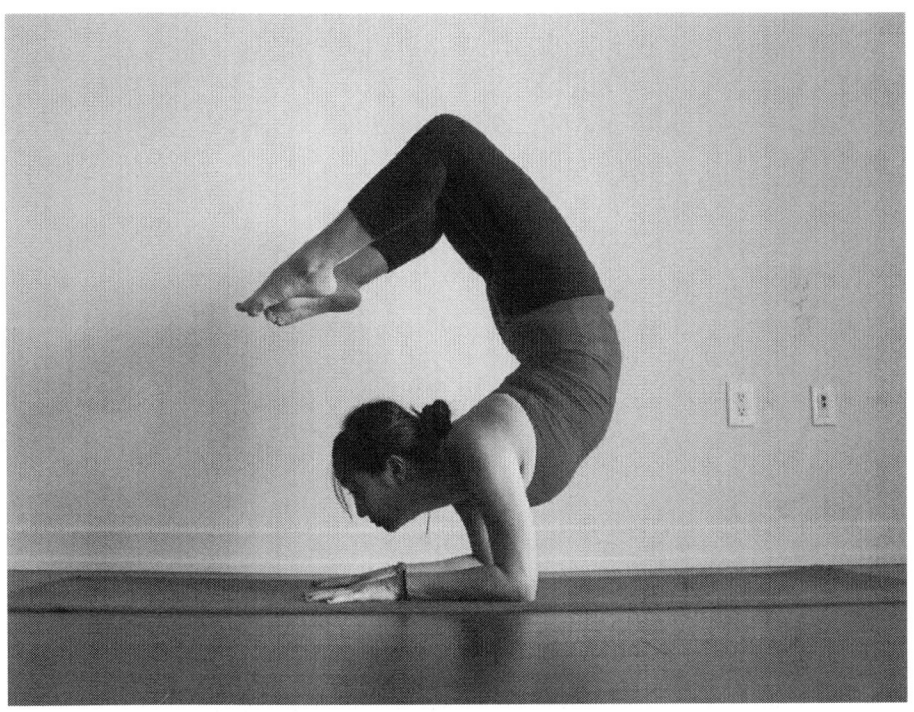

Photo Source: kharamkhare.com

63. PARSVA BAKASANA OR SIDE CROW POSE

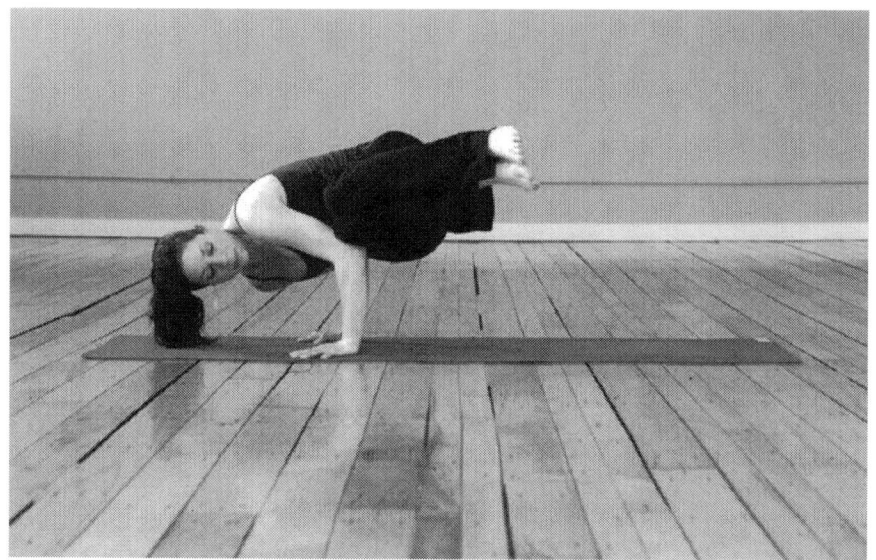

Photo Source: popsugar.com

64. DOWNWARD FACING DOG

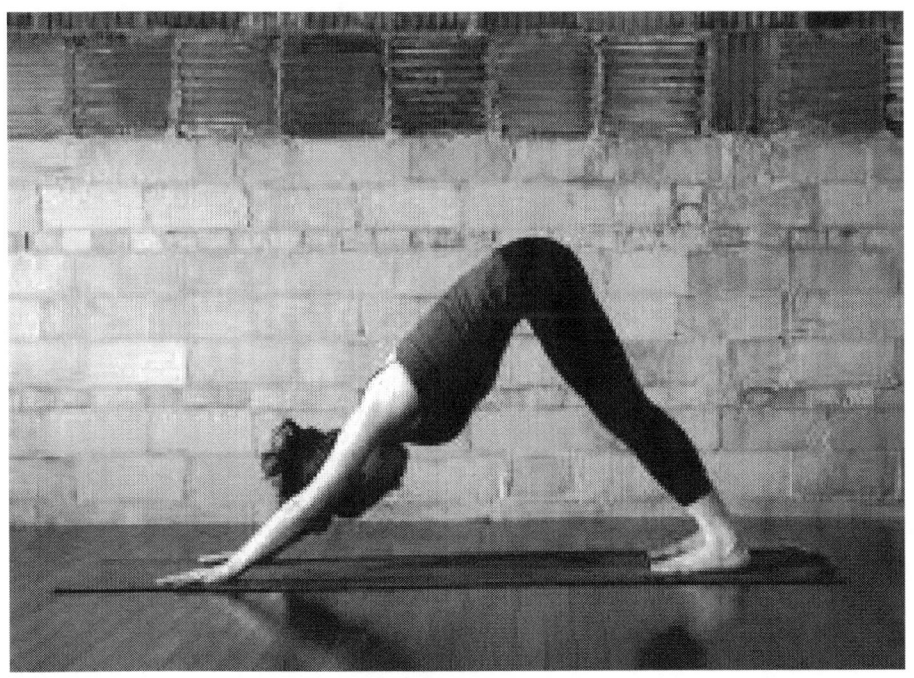

Photo Source: joycerey.com

CHAPTER 5

BACKBENDS

Backbends can be challenging poses, but they are amazing and they offer fantastic benefits, too. Backbends can generally relieve anxiety and stress, as well as increase your discipline, dedication, and mental strength.

Most backbends open up your chest. These poses also bring your spine to its natural flexion.

Backbends help increase your flexibility and relieve back and neck pain. These poses also increase your muscle strength.

Backbend poses stretch your abdominal muscles and increase the strength of your core. Backbends can be complex and intimidating, but practicing these poses can actually boost your courage and positive thinking. These poses help you go past your self-imposed limits.

Backbends are also proven to relieve insomnia and treat other sleeping disorders. These poses improve circulation, thus helping your body relax and sleep better.

65. CAMATKARASANA OR WILD THING

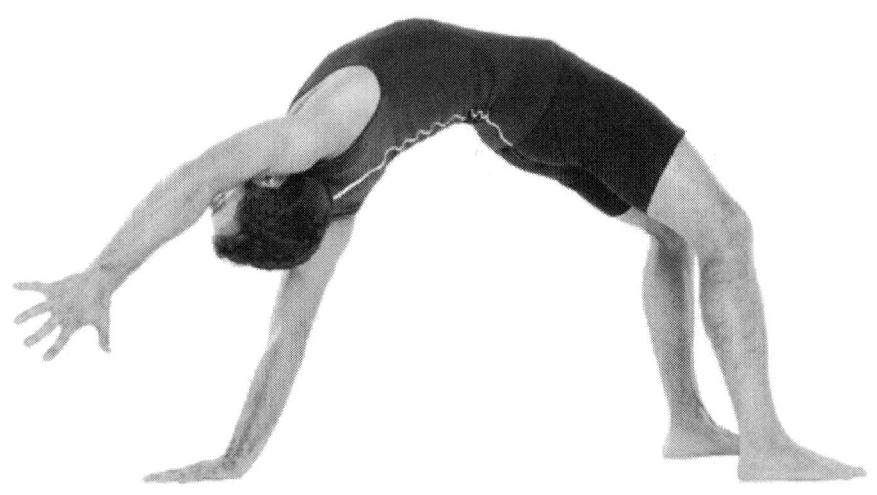

Photo Source: yogajournal.com

66. BOW POSE OR DHANURASANA

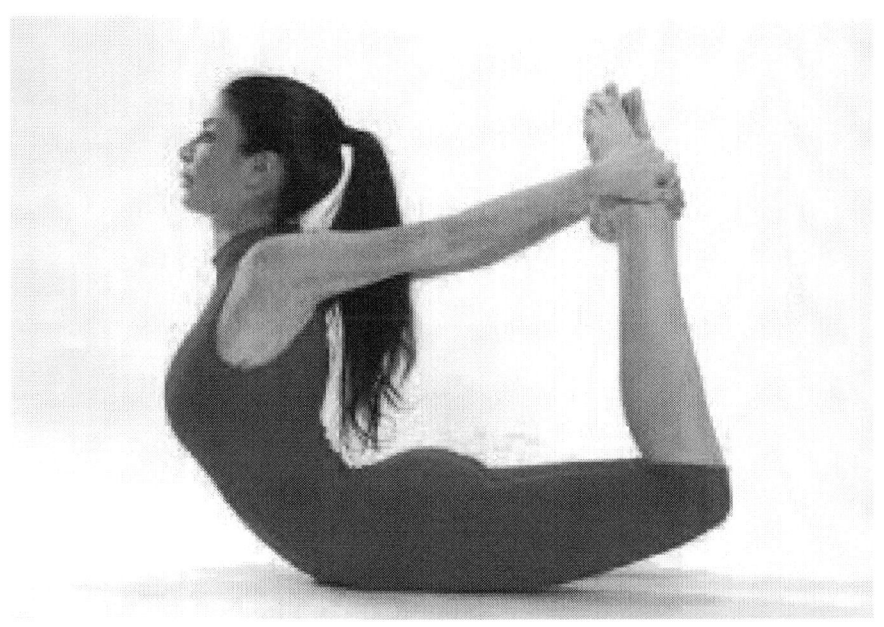

Photo Source: galleryhip.com

67. SETU BANDHA SARVANGASANA OR BRIDGE POSE

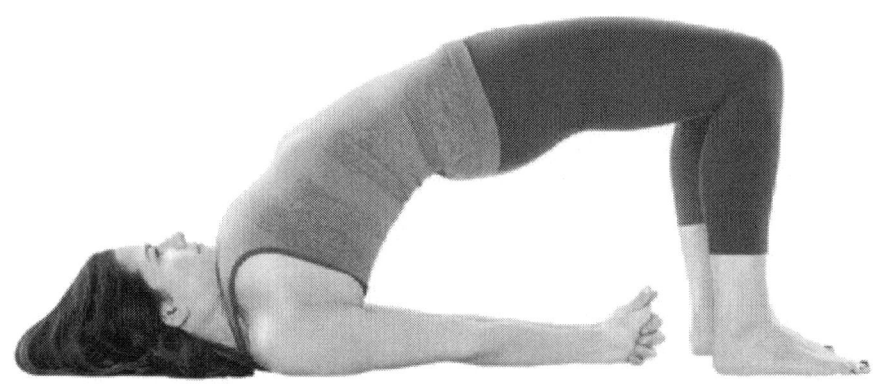

Photo Source: yogajournal.com

68. USTRASANA OR CAMEL POSE

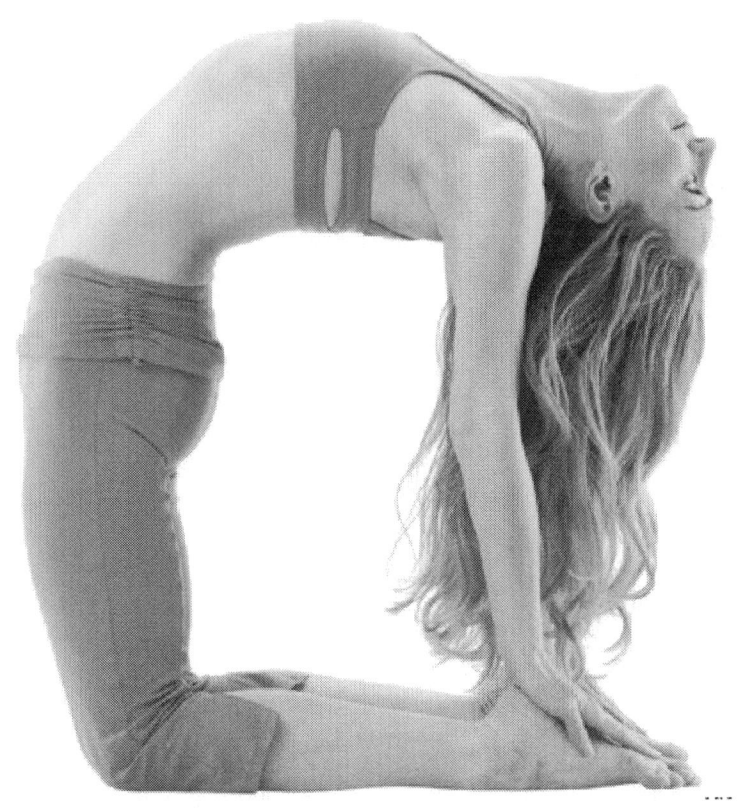

Photo Source: yogajournal.com

69. COBRA POSE OR BHUJANGASANA

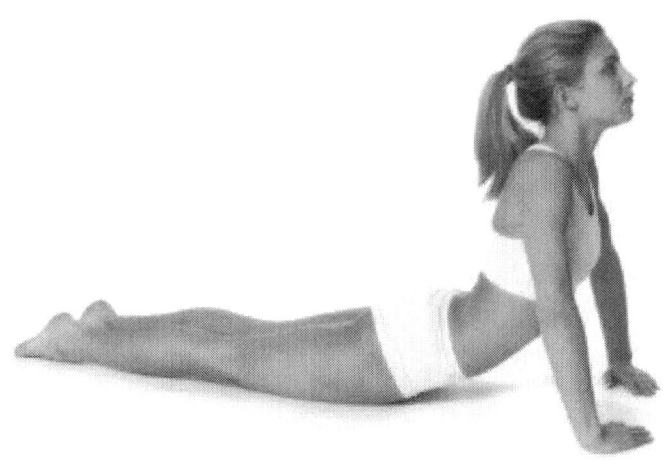

Photo Source: dailyperricone.com

70. FISH POSE OR MATSYASANA

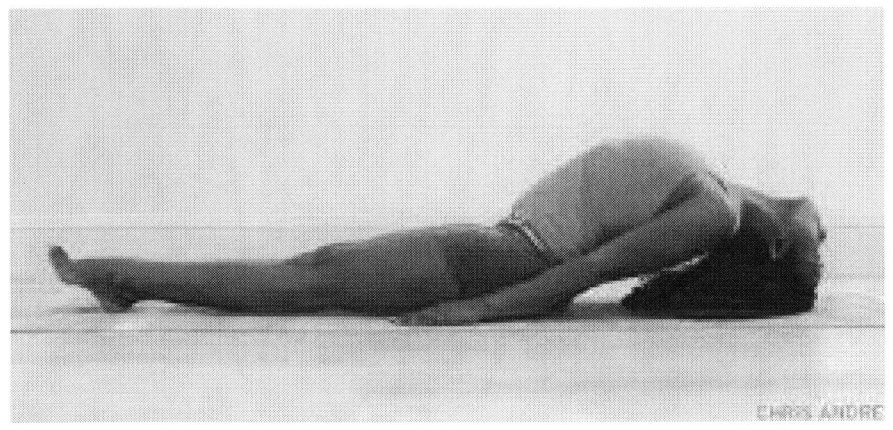

Photo Source: pixgood.com

71. COW POSE

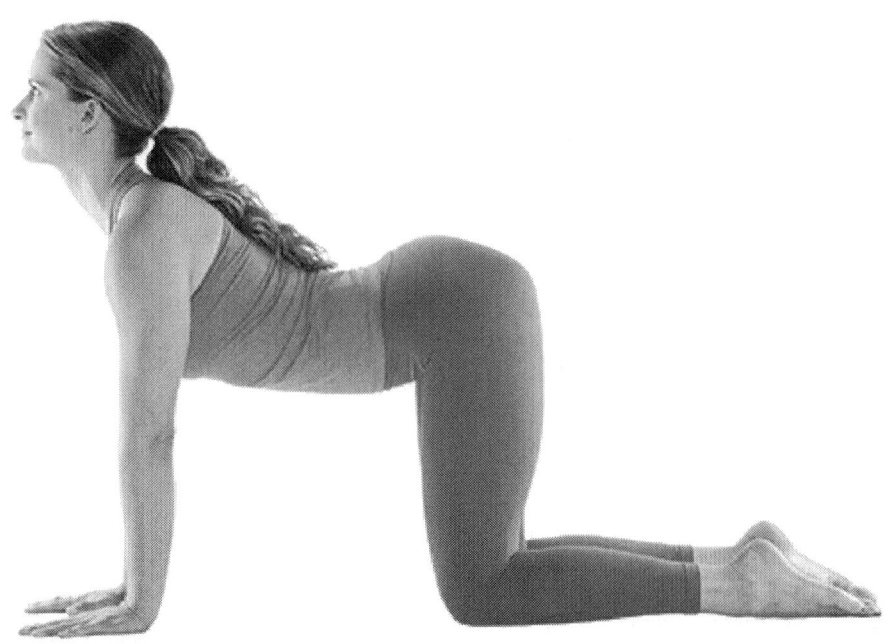

Photo Source: yogajournal.com

72. LOCUST POSE OR SALABHASANA

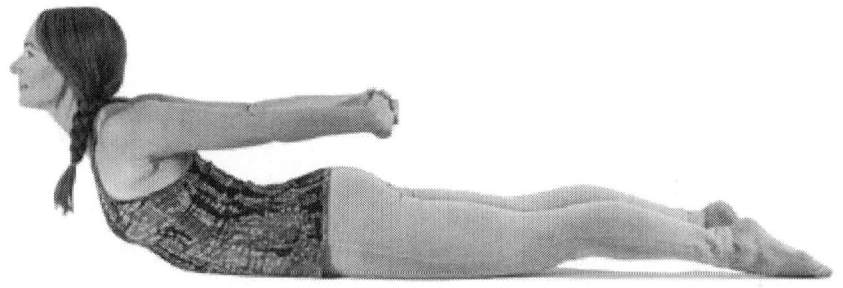

Photo Source: yogajournal.com

73. ARDHA SALABHASANA OR HALF LOCUST POSE

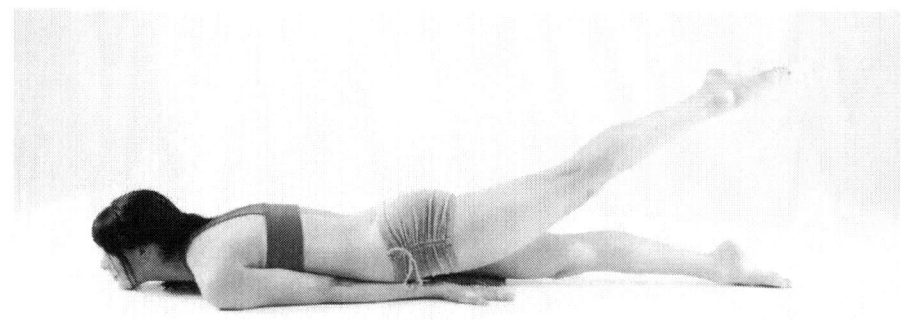

Photo Source: bikramlosangeles.com

74. FISH IN LOTUS POSE

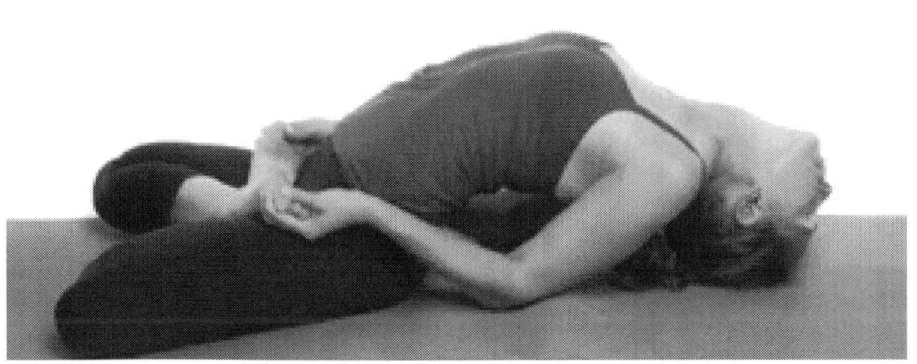

Photo Source: Fish in Lotus Pose

75. ONE-LEGGED KING PIGEON POSE OR EKA PADA RAJAKAPOTASANA

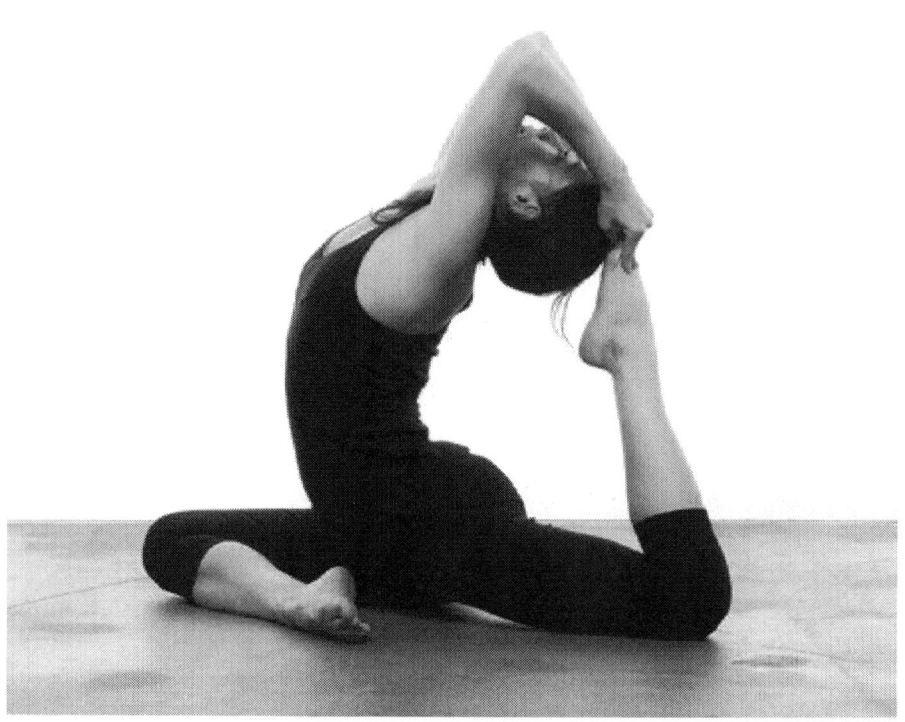

Photo Source: yogajournal.com

76. ONE-LEGGED KING PIGEON POSE II OR EKA PADA RAJAKAPOTASANA II

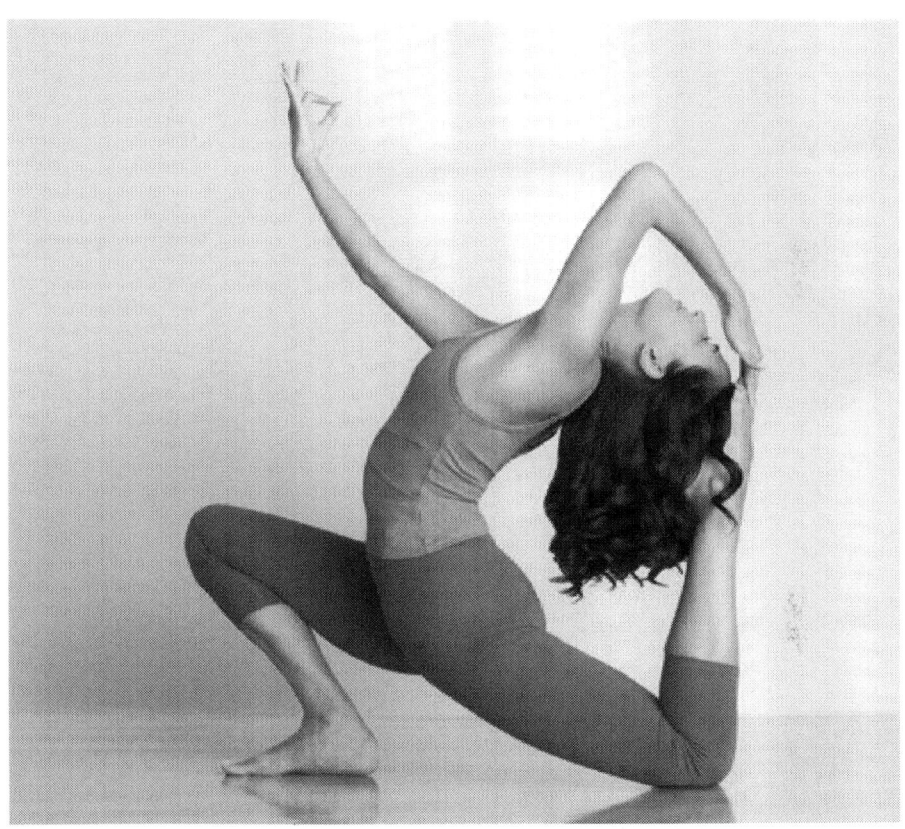

Photo Source: yogajournal.com

77. PIGEON POSE OR KAPOTASANA

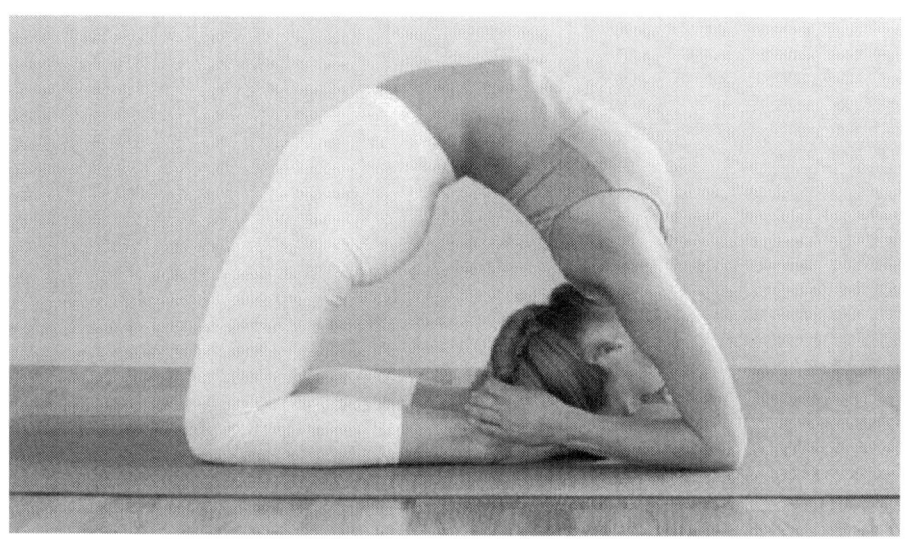

Photo Source: yogajournal.com

78. SPHINX POSE

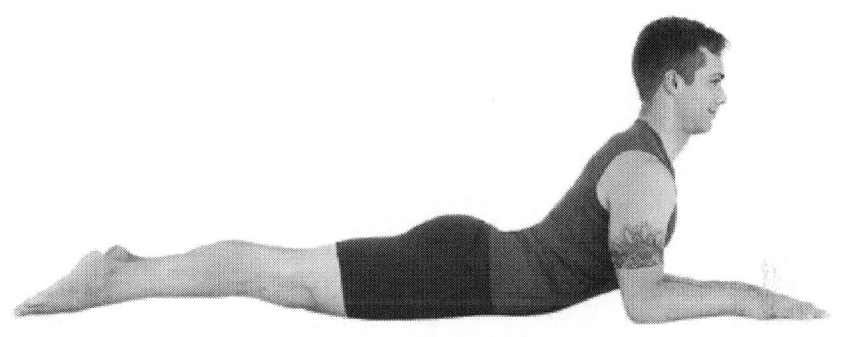

Photo Source: yogajournal.com

79. URDHVA DHANURASANA OR WHEEL POSE

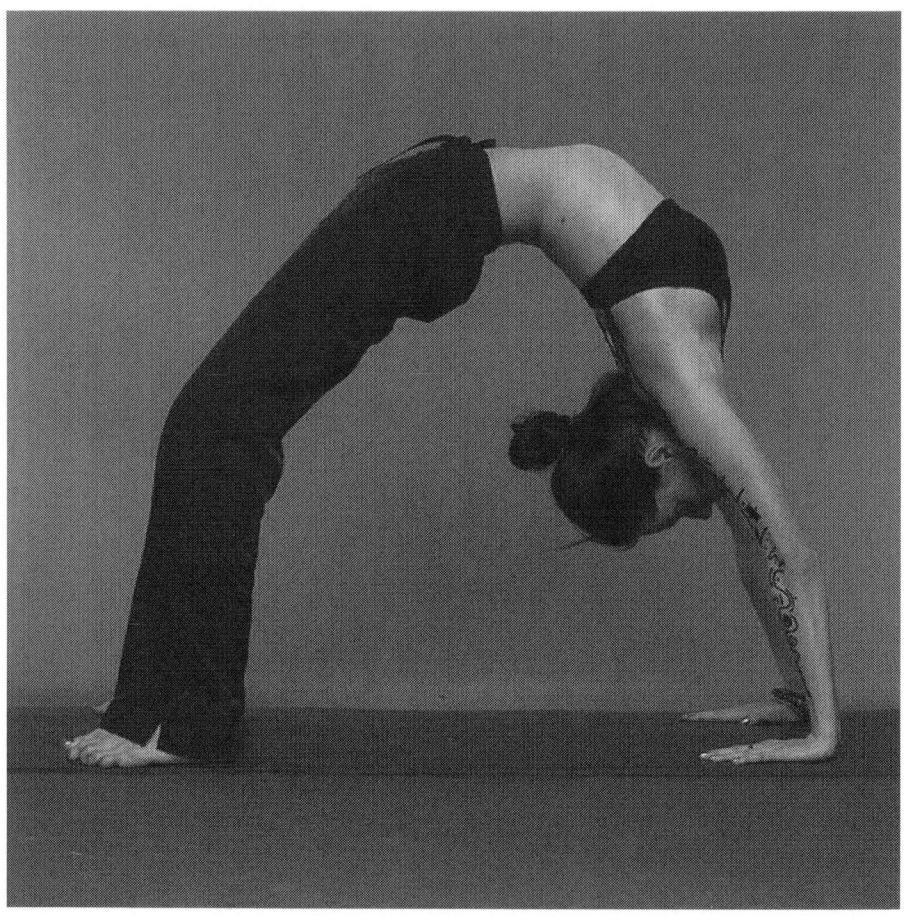

Photo Source: Wikipedia.org

80. URDHVA MUKHA SVANASANA OR UPWARD-FACING DOG POSE

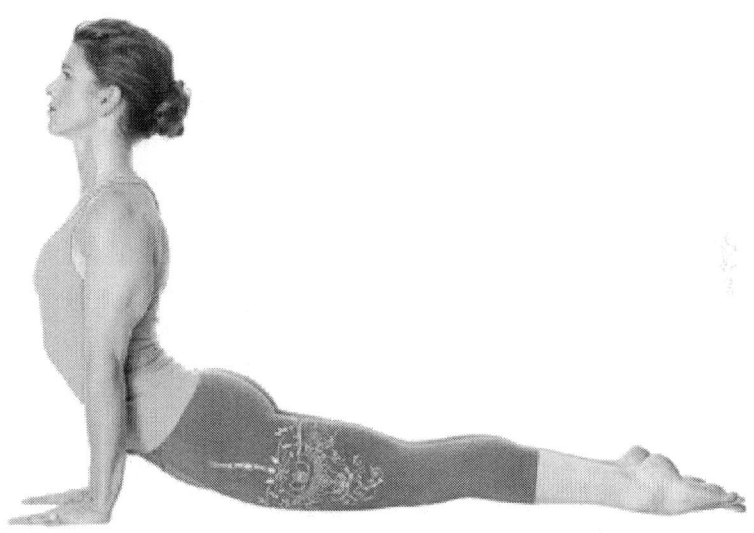

Photo Source: yogajournal.com

81. UPWARD FACING TWO-FOOT STAFF POSE OR DWI PADA VIPARITA DANDASANA

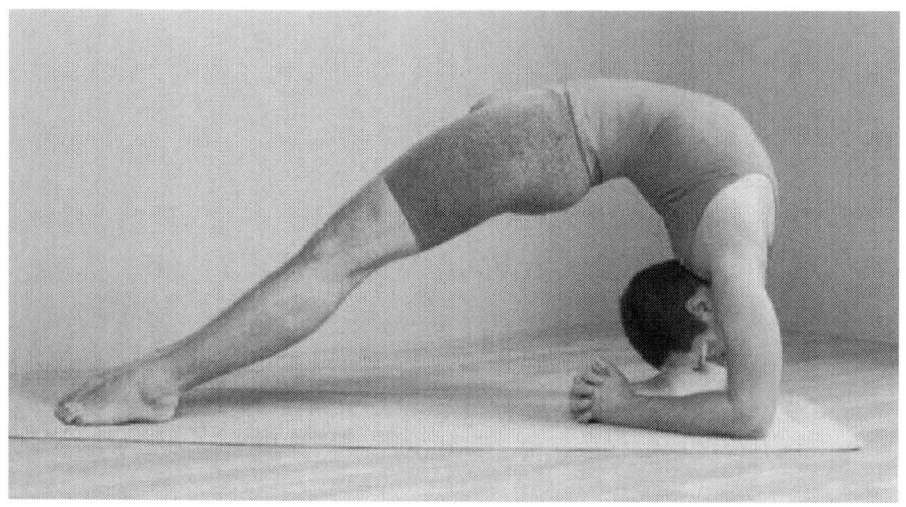

Photo Source: yogajournal.com

CHAPTER 6

OTHER POSES

There are actually more than 100,000 asanas or yoga poses. However, only a few numbers of the common poses are practiced in the West. In the next pages are the other poses that you should try. These poses are usually practiced in intermediate yoga classes.

These poses can help you lose more weight effectively. Since yoga improves cognitive functions and increases mindfulness, practicing these poses will help you make prudent choices regarding what you eat and drink. These poses also strengthen your immune system and increase your energy.

82. REVOLVED SIDE ANGLE OR PARIVRTTA PĀRŚVAKONASANA

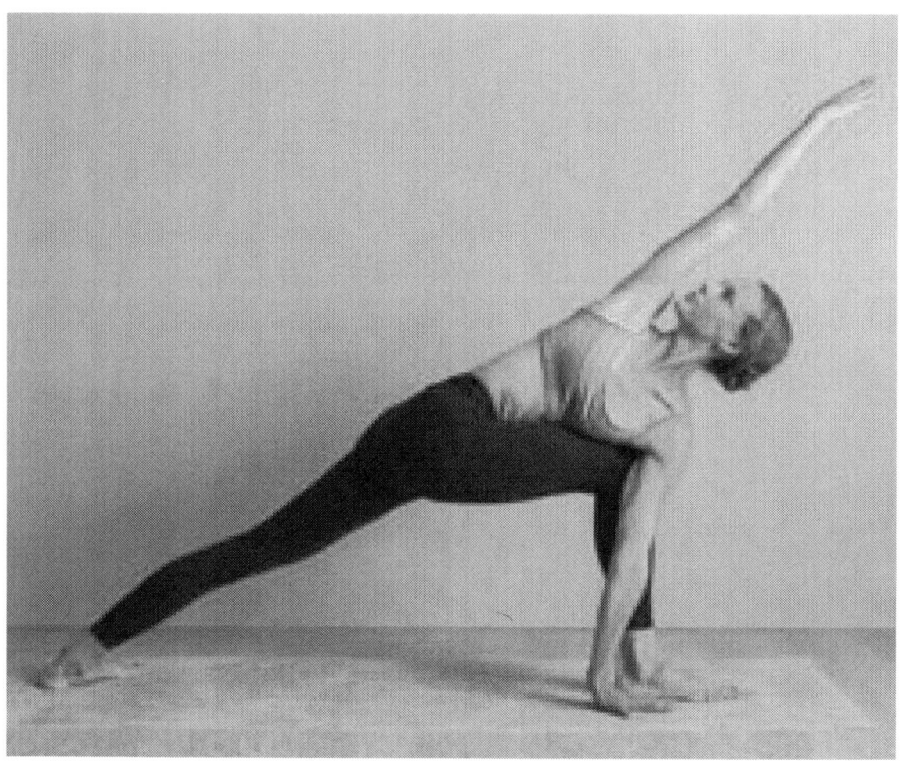

Photo Source: yogajournal.com

83. TORTOISE OR KŪRMĀSANA

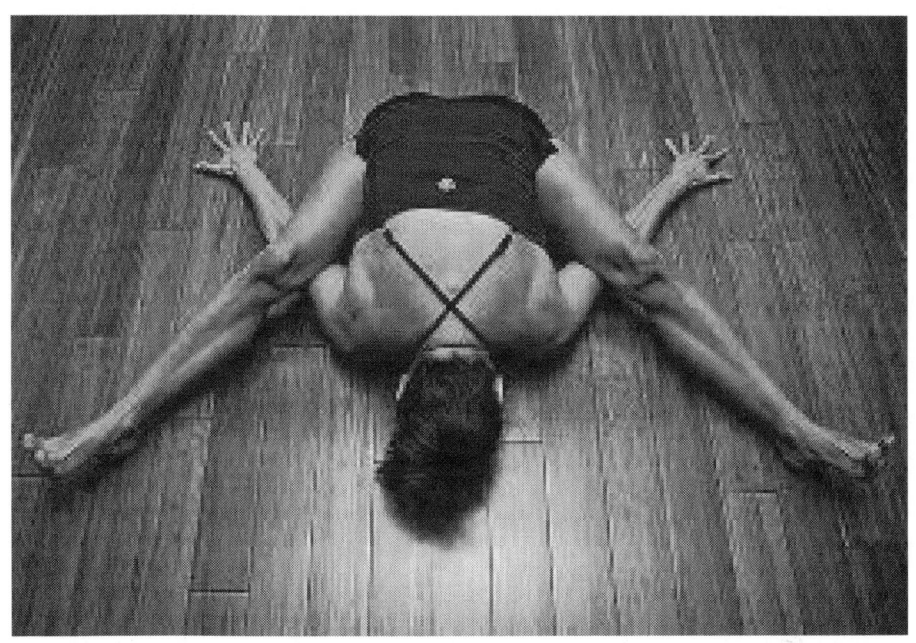

Photo Source: womenfitness.com

84. CROCODILE POSE OR MAKARĀSANA

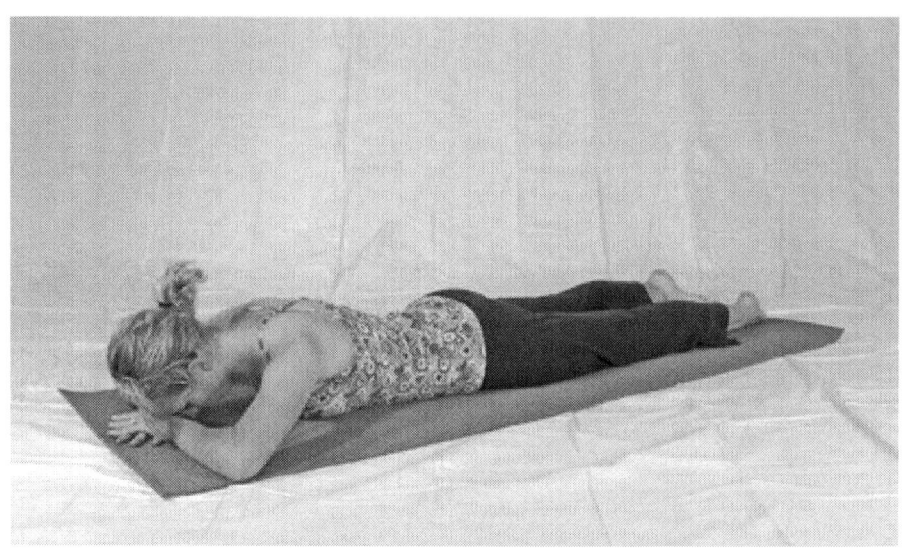

Photo Source: banyanbotanicals.com

85. NOOSE POSE OR PARYAṄKĀSANA

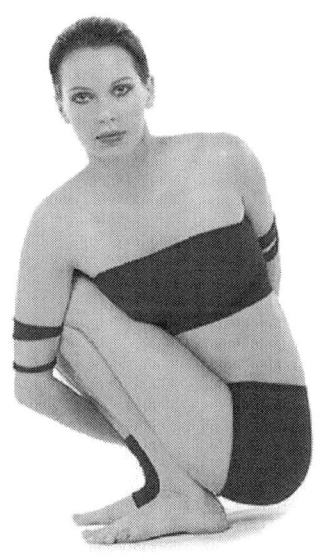

Photo Source: Wikipedia.org

86. LION POSE OR SIṀHĀSANA

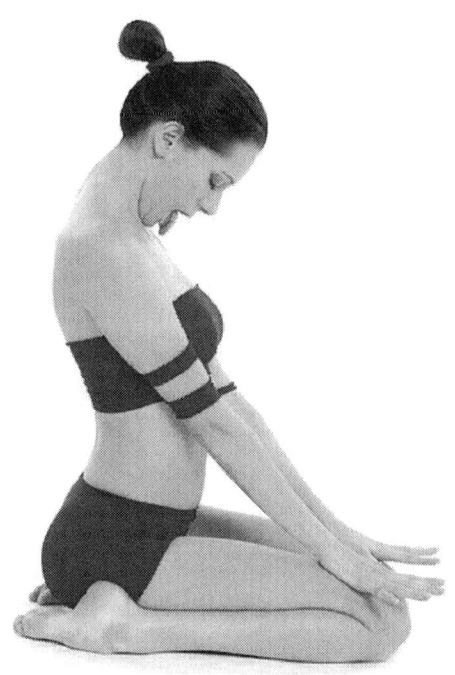

Photo Source: Wikipedia.org

87. CHILD'S POSE OR BĀLĀSANA

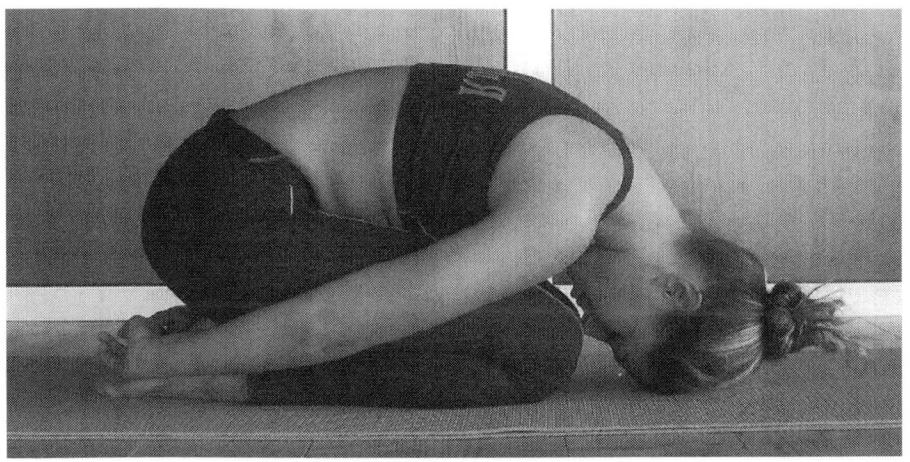

Photo Source: Wikipedia.org

88. PENDANT POSE OR LOLĀSANA

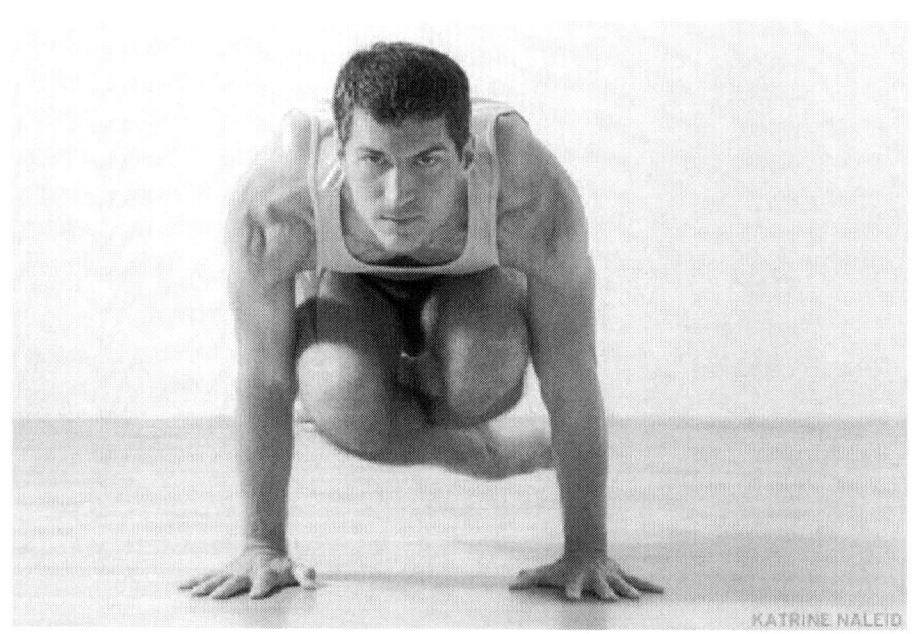

Photo Source: yogajournal.com

89. GARLAND POSE OR MĀLĀSANA

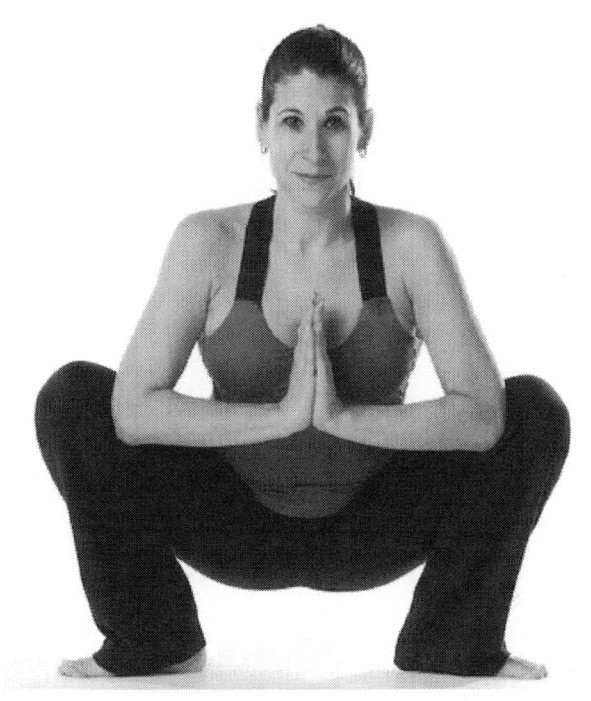

Photo Source: dietsinreview.com

90. EAR-PRESSING POSE OR KARṆAPĪḌĀSANA

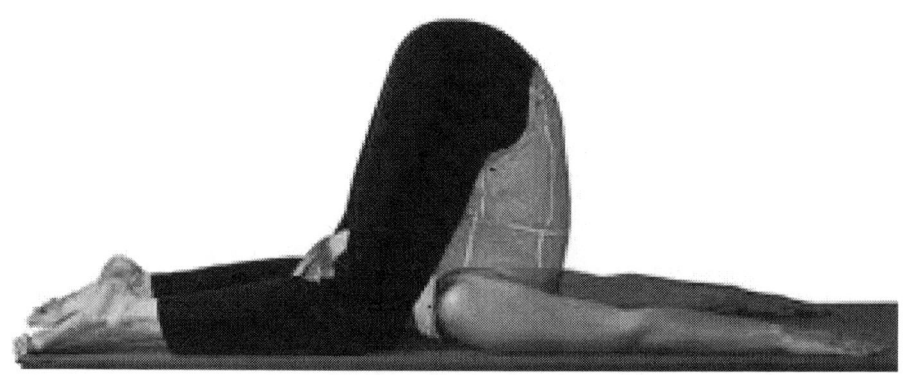

Photo Source: fitho.in

91. BELLY REVOLVING POSTURE OR JAṬHARAPARIVARTANĀSANA

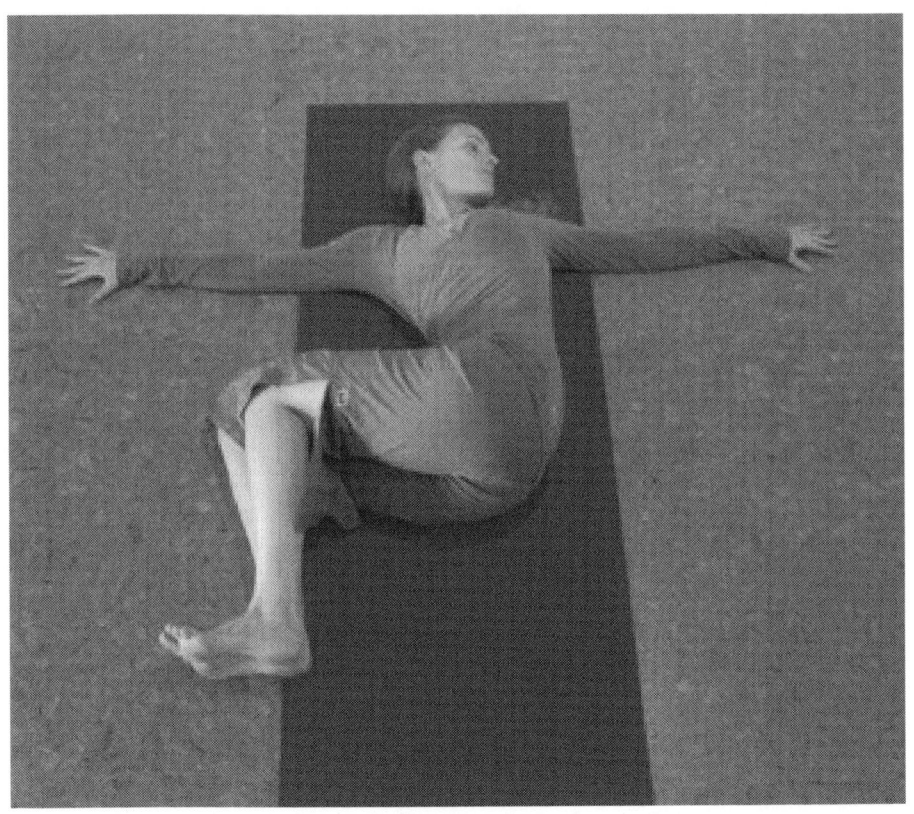

Photo Source: fitho.in

92. FETUS POSE OR GARBHĀSANA

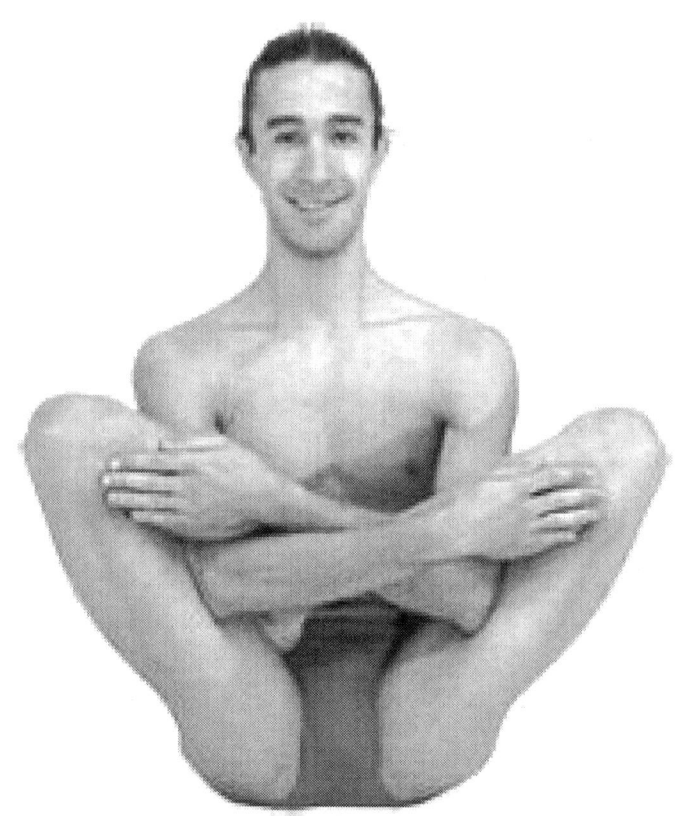

Photo Source: Wikipedia.org

93. HAPPY BABY POSE

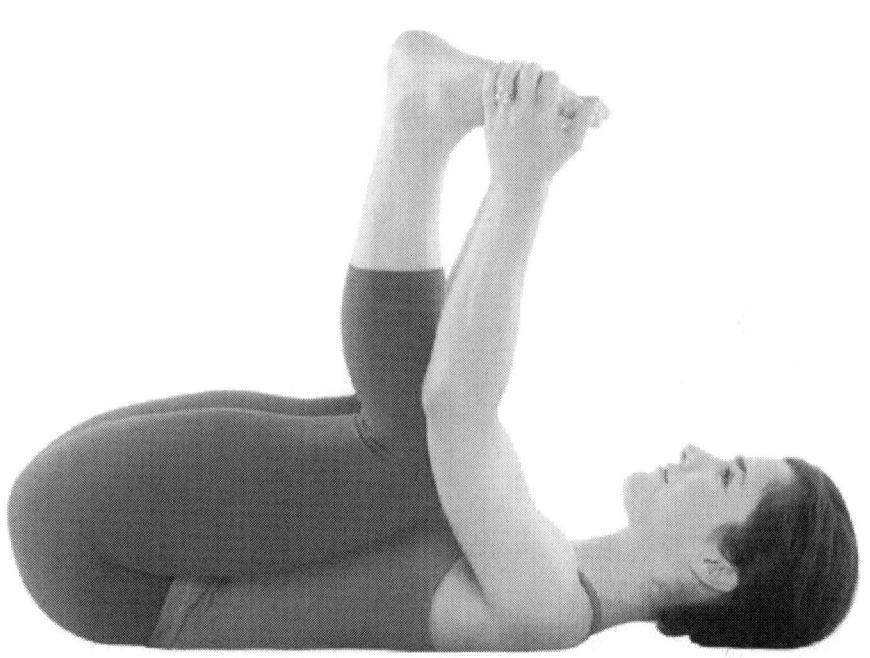

Photo Source: yogajournal.com

94. CORPSE POSE

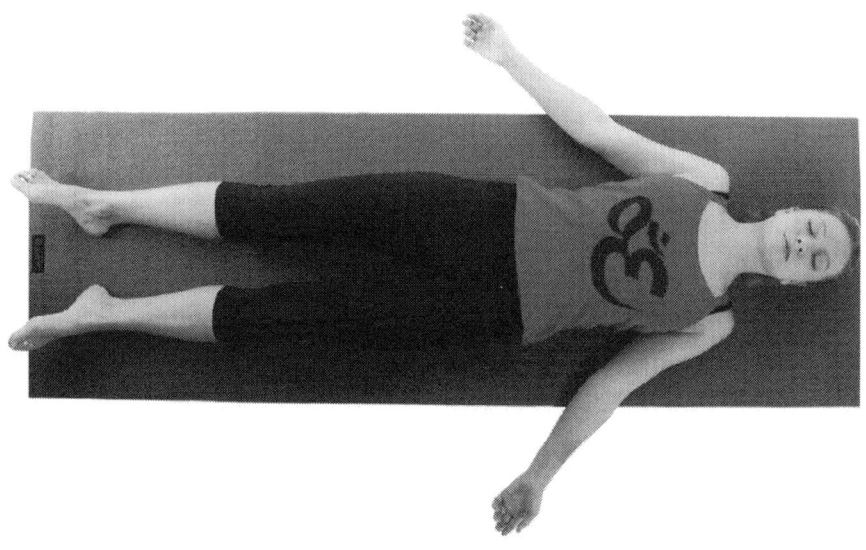

Photo Source: yogaily.com

95. RABBIT POSE OR SASANGASANA

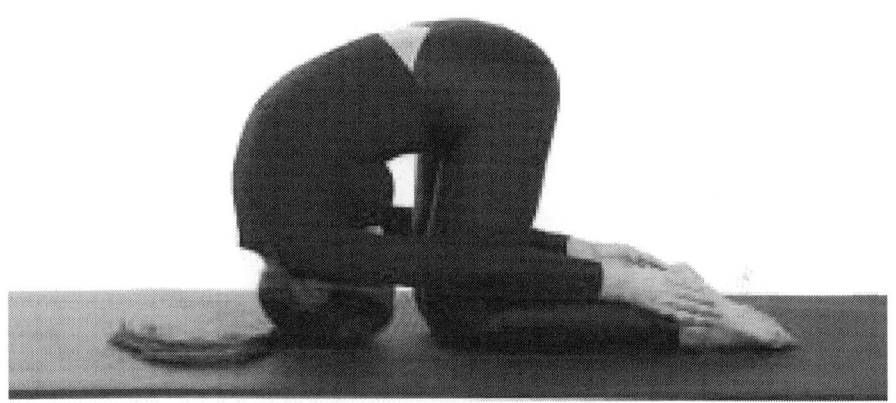

Photo Source: lovemyyoga.com

96. ZEN POSE OR SUPTAVAJRĀSANA

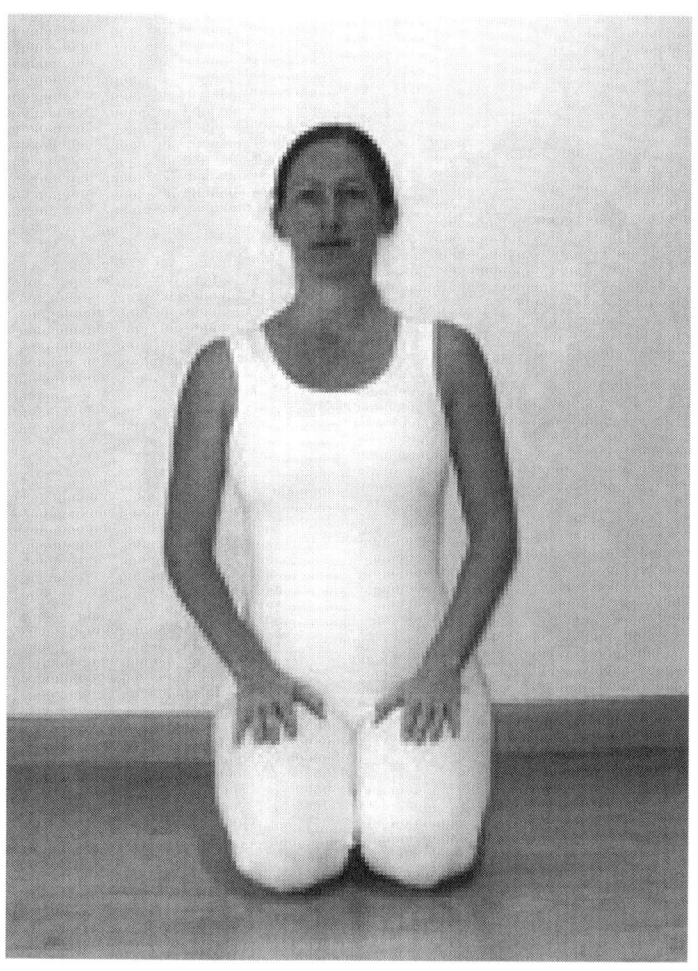

Photo Source: yogalearningcenter.com

97. GODDESS POSE

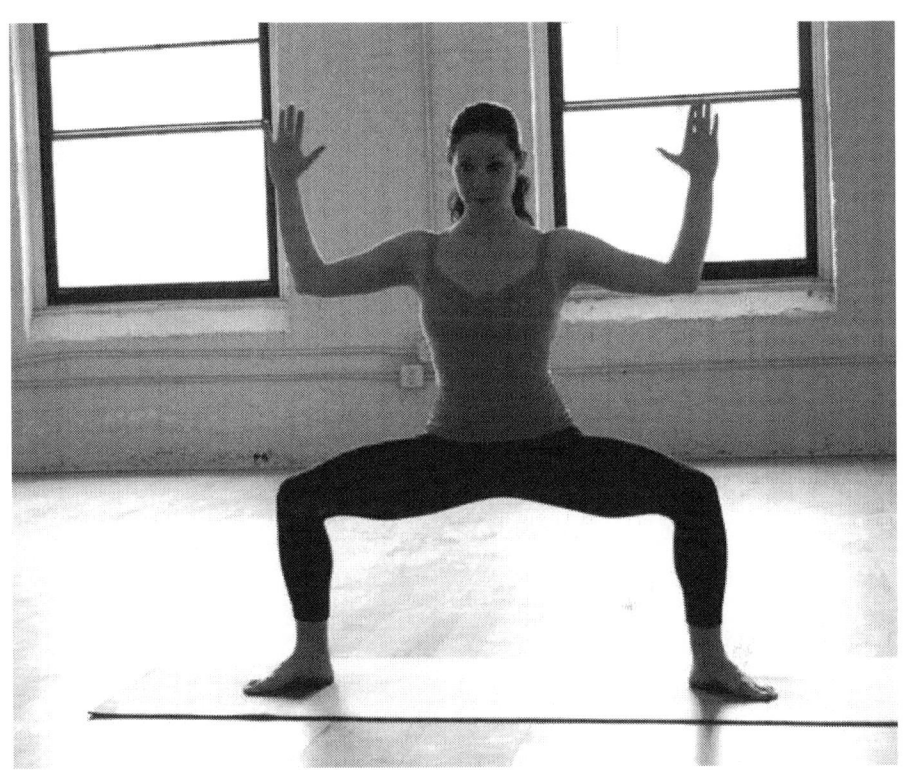

Photo Source: goddess.com

98. VATAYANASANA OR HORSE POSE

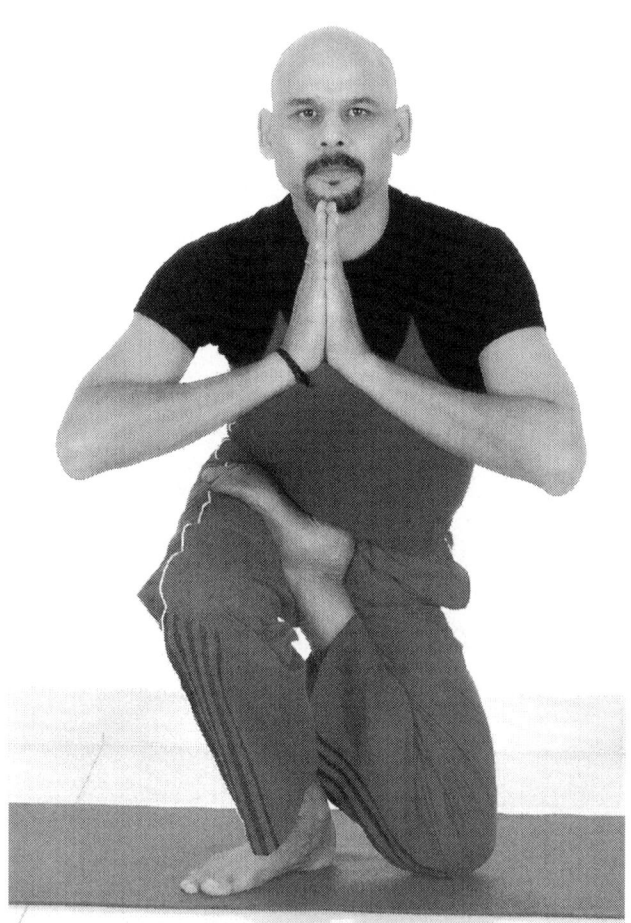

Photo Source: my.yoga-vidya.org

99. PEACOCK FEATHER POSE WITH LEGS IN PADMASANA/ELBOW BALANCE

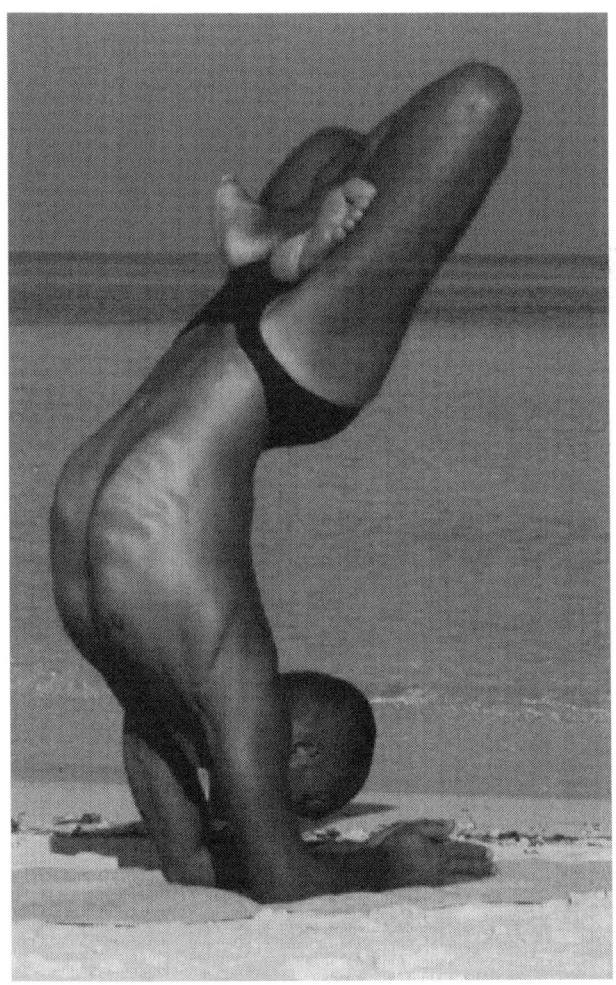

Photo Source: Wikipedia.org

100. RECLINING BOUND ANGLE OR SUPTABADDHAKONĀSANA

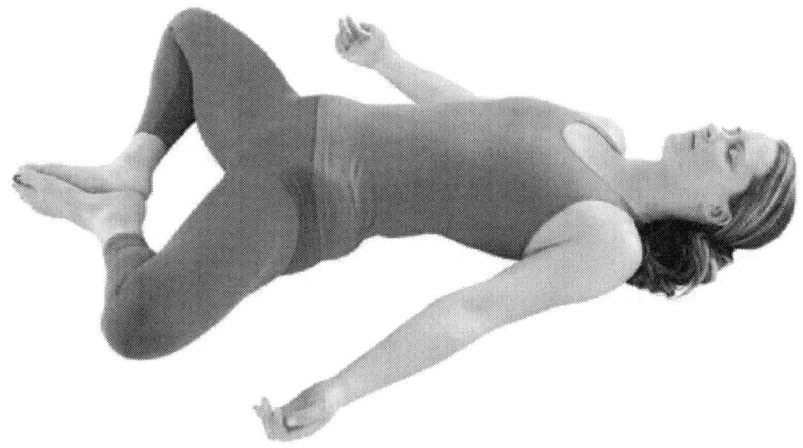

Photo Source: yogajournal.com

CHAPTER 7

SAFETY TIPS

When you are practicing yoga, your safety should be your highest priority. Here are some safety tips that will prevent you from getting injured while practicing yoga:

Discuss your physical condition with your instructor.

It is important to discuss your physical conditions and limitations with your yoga instructor before you begin. You also need to let your yoga instructor know if you are pregnant.

Do not compete with others.

Remember that yoga is not a competition. Do not compare your performance and abilities with those of other people. Do not force yourself to keep up with other people. Assume each pose as gently as you can so that you won't strain yourself.

Stay within your limits.

It is important to discover your physical limits and to stay within those limits. This will keep you from getting injured. Remember to listen to your body.

Do not forget to do warm-up exercises before your yoga class.

It is important to prepare your muscles for the tedious yoga poses.

Thus, it is important to do warm-up exercises before you begin your workout routine.

Wear loose clothing.

To ensure that you can assume each pose without exerting more effort than what is necessary, it is important that you wear comfortable clothing. This will allow you to move more freely.

Pick the right yoga class.

There are different types of yoga, so you have to pick the one that is right for you.

- Hatha Yoga – This type of yoga teaches the different yoga postures. It is best for beginners.

- Ashtanga Yoga – This is generally an aerobic exercise since it is fast-paced and rigorous. Ashtanga yoga repeats the same postures in the same order over and over.

- Vinyasa Yoga – This type of yoga practice is known for its fluidity. The movement from one pose to another is smooth and effortless.

- Restorative Yoga – This type of yoga practice is used to relax and soothe the nerves. Restorative yoga is rejuvenating and it helps relieve stress and anxiety.

- Bikram Y0ga – This practice is done in a heated room. This type of yoga is best for weight loss.

- Iyengar Yoga – This type of practice is meticulous. Many props are used in an Iyengar yoga class to ensure proper alignment of the body.

Yoga is a great exercise that can offer tremendous health benefits. Nonetheless, it is important to use the right pose and to choose the type of practice that is most ideal for you.

CONCLUSION

Thank you again for downloading this book!

I hope this book was able to help you get acquainted with the different yoga poses.

The next step is to apply what you have learned in this book to change your life. Yoga has tremendous physical and mental health benefits. It strengthens your mind and your body. Yoga also helps keep your body fit, too. Yoga is fun, light, and challenging at the same time.

Also, it is important to consult your doctor before trying any of the poses featured in this book. If you are a beginner, it is best to start your yoga practice under the supervision of a certified yoga teacher.

Finally, if you enjoyed this book, please take the time to share your thoughts and post a positive review on Amazon. It'd be greatly appreciated!

Thank you and good luck!

13639245R00069

Printed in Great Britain
by Amazon.co.uk, Ltd.,
Marston Gate.